Biopsy Decoded

A Patient's Guide to Modern Biopsies, Diagnostic Accuracy, and Peace of Mind

First Edition

Tesfu Hailu, MD, FCAP, FASCP, FASDP
Board Certified Anatomic Pathologist and Dermatopathologist

All medical illustrations were produced exclusively for the author by Dr. Naduni Prabhathi, physician and medical illustrator. The author holds full copyright via a fee-for-service transfer.

All flowcharts were prepared by the author using the open-source mermaid.live platform. Grammatical corrections, brainstorming, source searches, and editorial refinements were performed in Microsoft 360 with the assistance of Copilot, Claude, and Gemini AI tools.

Hardcover ISBN: 979-8-9959260-2-3
Paperback ISBN: 979-8-9959260-0-9
eBook ISBN: 979-8-9959260-1-6

Preface: The Quiet Art of Medicine My Journey to Pathology

The hands often find their purpose long before the heart catches up.

For as long as I can remember, I was the boy with the restless hands. To my family and neighbors, I was the tinkerer child who could conjure playthings out of the mundane, weaving toys from the jagged remains of rusted barbed wire. I remember kids lining up, waiting with bated breath as I fashioned one crude, rustic wire-wheel after another.

My grandmother, however, always watched my crafty obsession with a mix of scorn and terror. She always branded me 'Ketkatch', a derogatory Amharic slur for an unskilled metalsmith, and spat out a dark prophecy whenever she saw me tinkering: "One day, he'll stumble upon an unexploded Italian bomb and lose a limb". To her, my hands were flirting with disaster; to me, they were simply having fun, busy building a world from scrap. The hands often find their purpose long before the heart catches up.

In my early years as a medical student and later as a General Practitioner in Ethiopia, my hands were my primary interface with the world. I took a quiet, rhythmic pride in the clean work of minor outpatient surgical procedures. There is a specific, meditative cadence to it: the subtle tactile resistance of tissue, the quiet weight of a patient's trust placed in a student or intern, and the deep, silent satisfaction of a perfectly placed suture.

My mentors noticed it early, often remarking on my skills. I carried myself with the quiet confidence of a man who believed his destiny was written in manual dexterity and an obsession with the fine ar chitecture of human anatomy.

At that time, if you had told me I would one day abandon the scalpel, I would have laughed. I loved the performance of surgery, the immediate, visible impact of a procedure well-executed. But beneath that love for the doing rested a hidden deeper, more artistic scientific hunger: a fascination with the why. I didn't just want only to repair the body; I also wanted to decode the silent, microscopic language it spoke.

The North American Trial

Migrating to Canada was a rebirth, but one paved with the 'cold', hard reality of the immigrant experience. I was half a world away from home, thrown into a chaotic mix of career anxiety and a cultural shock. I poured my soul into the Canadian medical licensing exams, crossing every t and dotting every i. I passed them all. Yet the gate remained locked.

In Canada, residency spots for international graduates were a vanishingly small target, not due to exclusion, but because a country of such vast geography has a disproportionately small population and limited hospital infrastructure. Even Canadian medical graduates sometimes must travel to the United States for residency training.

Persistence, however, is a physician's best trait. I turned my sights toward the United States, challenging the USMLE exams one by one, still driven by the singular goal of becoming a surgeon. I lived in a state of constant motion, studying, testing, planning, until a single afternoon of curiosity changed the trajectory of my life forever.

The Vision in Pink and Blue

While plotting my path for getting into a surgery residency program, a stray thought crossed my mind: What is my fallback plan? I began working through a list of various specialties, ranking and moving down the list until I hit Pathology. My only exposure in histopathology had been the basic science courses - Anatomy, Histology, and Pathology. I remember loving them with a strange, fierce passion, spending weekends, Christmases, and summer holidays in anatomy dissection rooms and histology labs, hunched over a microscope while others were away on vacation. Living with my parents across from the medical school where they both worked made this immersion possible.

Driven by a sudden, electric impulse, I decided to put my love for the basic sciences to the ultimate test. I wanted to see if the raw, intellectual curiosity I'd carried since medical school, could survive the high-octane, high-tech crucible of North American medicine. With nothing but a sense of mission, I marched into the Department of Laboratory Medicine at St. Paul's Hospital in the heart of downtown Vancouver, ready to find out if my future lay under a lens.

I must have radiated a certain charming desperation, because my fervent pitch to see a real-world Canadian pathologist actually worked. A kind pathologist, perhaps sensing the genuine fire behind my questions, didn't just give me directions, she invited me into her world. Sit here, she said, gesturing toward the observer's seat of her towering, multi-headed microscope.

She slid a glass slide onto the stage. As I leaned into the eyepieces, the hospital walls, the exams, and the stress of the previous years simply vanished. Before me was a biopsy of a human liver, stained with Hematoxylin and Eosin (H&E).

It was a masterpiece. I saw the artistic rendering of the cells, the delicate contrast of pinks and purples, the architectural flow of the hexagonal lobules. It was the most beautiful thing I had ever seen.

Then, she performed a small act that felt like a magician's reveal. She swapped the slide for a Trichrome stained one.

Suddenly, the world turned blue, red, and purple. The vibrant, deep cobalt of the connective tissue against the cellular background was so visceral it felt like a physical blow. Goosebumps erupted across my arms. My eyes welled with tears as a realization crashed over me: This is it.

In that moment, the performance of surgery felt distant and hollow compared to the absolute truth of the microscope. I realized that the rest of my life would be spent here, immersed in this artistic, diagnostic rendering of the human anatomic histology.

I left that room a different man. I was no longer an aspiring surgeon. I was a pathologist in conception.

The 120 Letters

The epiphany was beautiful, but the timing was disastrous. It was the end of May when the results for my USMLE Step 3 have come heralding my success. The National Resident Matching Program was over. The seats were filled. The doors were shut. Conventional wisdom said to wait another year, to sit on the sidelines while my passion cooled.

But I thought of the human element. What if someone who matched couldn't show up? Life happens! What if a seat was empty and a program was desperate?

I turned to the Green Book, the directory of every residency program in the country. I digitized all the email addresses of approximately 120 Pathology programs across the continental United States. I wrote a cover letter that didn't just list my credentials but told my story. I attached my CV along with, as freshly wed, a photograph of myself with my beautiful wife, Hiwot Adane, I wanted them to see the family, the person, and the dream behind the application.

Using an SMTP automation tool that I wrote myself (I'm a self-taught client-server application developer), I sent 120 individual, personalized emails. Then, I waited.

The 20-Minute Miracle

I had braced myself for the long, agonizing silence of a reply, a void of weeks or months where hope usually goes to wither.

Instead, the silence lasted barely twenty minutes when the responses began to arrive in a rapid, digital succession. My inbox was transformed into a hub of activity, with twenty-three residency programs expressing a combination of intrigue and genuine surprise. The program directors were impressed, not only by the strength of my credentials but by the unprecedented initiative it took to reach out at such a critical juncture.

Most of the responses were encouraging, inviting me to join their ranks for the upcoming cycle. But amidst the digital noise, one message stood out with singular clarity: an email from Dr. Cheryl Hanau at Hahnemann University Hospital in Philadelphia!

They had a rare, off-cycle opening, a crack in the door that shouldn't have been there. I didn't wait. I picked up the phone and called Dr. Hanau immediately.

Within minutes of our conversation, the academic world felt personal again. I was struck not only by her professionalism, but also by her profound attention to me as a person, as a human being, and an unmistakable compassionate mentorship spirit that radiated even through the phone line.

In that short conversation, the uncertainty of my journey evaporated. I wasn't just looking for a residency anymore; I had found a home. I was sold.

I moved to Philadelphia, stepped into the hospital, and began my training journey to the career I was born for: **Pathologist!**

Tesfu Hailu, MD, FCAP, FASDP, FASCP
Board-Certified Anatomic Pathologist and Dermatopathologist

Why This Book Exists

Every year, tens of millions of people hear a single word that instantly changes the way they breathe, sleep, and think: Biopsy.

For most patients, that word carries fear, uncertainty, and a sense that something important has been set in motion, often without a clear understanding of what is actually happening or why. The space between the procedure and the results can feel like a long, uncomfortable silence filled with questions.

This book exists to fill that silence with understanding.

As a pathologist, I examine the tissue that carries answers to some of the most important questions patients ever face. I know how much meaning is packed into each word of a pathology report, and how confusing those words can feel when you are reading them without a guide. I also know that fear thrives in mystery, while understanding creates steadiness and confidence.

This book was written to pull back the curtain.

It explains what a biopsy truly is, how and why it is done, what happens to tissue after it leaves your body, how diagnoses are made at the microscopic level, and how to read your pathology report with better understanding. It is designed to turn technical language into understandable concepts, without stripping away accuracy or honesty.

Most importantly, this book exists to remind you that the pathologist is constantly aware that behind every biopsy slide is a person, and behind every diagnosis is a careful, deliberate process aimed at finding the truth so the right treatment can follow.

If you are awaiting results, preparing for a biopsy, reviewing a report, or simply trying to understand what a loved one is going through, this book is meant to be a steady companion. It does not promise answers before the microscope does. But it promises transparency, context, and respect for your intelligence and your humanity.

A biopsy is an act of courage.

Understanding it should never feel out of reach.

Disclaimer

This book is intended for educational purposes only. The content in this book is designed to help readers better understand biopsies, diagnostic processes, and general procedural concepts. It is not a substitute for professional medical advice, diagnosis, or treatment.

Every individual's medical situation is unique, and biopsy findings must be interpreted by qualified healthcare professionals who have full access to a patient's history, imaging, laboratory results, and clinical presentation. Do not use the information in this book to make decisions about your health or to delay seeking medical care.

Always consult a licensed physician or other qualified healthcare provider with any questions regarding a biopsy result, medical condition, or treatment plan. Never disregard or delay professional medical advice because of something you have read in this book.

While every effort has been made to ensure accuracy, medicine and pathology evolve, and information may change over time. The author and publisher assume no responsibility for errors, omissions, or outcomes resulting from the use of this material.

Table of Contents

Introduction

Every slide that crosses my desk and lands on my microscope stage is a world of its own, a kaleidoscope landscape of pinks, blues, reds, and purples that hold the answers to a patient's concern.

Looking through a microscope at a tissue sample can feel like staring at a piece of abstract art. To a pathologist, it is a language. We are the medical world's hidden detectives, translating the apparent chaos of cellular patterns into a definitive diagnosis.

People often ask me how I can look at a piece of tissue for only few seconds and know exactly what is wrong. The truth is, pathology isn't just a science job; it's also an art. It's about pattern recognition, rapid scanning, and knowing exactly what out of place looks like.

I remember once when I was a pathology resident at Hahnemann. I wanted to buy a specific fountain pen as a gift for a friend. Before heading out, I did my research, I Googled exactly which types were popular in his native country, which ones his generation favored, and why. I narrowed it down to one specific model, printed out a picture of it, and memorized every detail.

I walked into a famous fountain pen store in New York that was packed with glass cases and polished wooden shelves, housing nothing other than different varieties and types of fountain pens, ball-pens, and everything in between. In every direction, there were rows upon rows of fountain pens glinting under the lights. I was greeted by a woman seated at the center of the store, who welcomed me with an easy warmth that felt instantly genuine.

I stepped in and quickly scanned the walls, left, right, and center. Within about 30 seconds, I knew the specific fountain pen I wanted wasn't there.

As I began to quietly back out of the store, she interrupted me. "You look like you are overwhelmed, she said."

I laughed sarcastically. "No, I'm not overwhelmed. You don't have the kind of fountain pen I'm looking for."

She laughed and said, "I have every type of fountain pen. There is no way you could glance at my store for few seconds and tell me I don't have what you're looking for!"

At this point, I pulled the printed paper out of my back pocket and showed her the picture. She looked at it with awe, her eyes going wide, and she said, "Oh my goodness... you are right. I don't have this one."

She was stunned and genuinely curious how I was able to quickly know that her store doesn't have what I was looking for.

I looked at her and said My lady, I know how to scan. I am being trained to see!

Her intrigue and curiosity increased. She asked what I did for a living, I told her that I was a Pathologist in training.

That fountain pen shop in New York was no different than a biopsy slide. When I look at a slide, I am looking at thousands of cells, a store full of information. But because I know exactly what I am looking for, I can scan through the shelves of cells and tissue and spot the one thing that doesn't belong there or the something that is missing.

This book is about that process. It's about how we see, how we catch the imposters hiding in plain sight, and how you, as a patient, can understand the report that comes from behind the microscope.

Part I

The Art of Naming the Unknown

Chapter 1

The Weight of a Word

A biopsy is an act of courage.

Understanding it should never feel out of reach.

In the quiet ecosystem of a hospital, some words carry the momentum of action, while others pulse with hope. Surgery sounds like a solution; Treatment sounds like a path forward. But Biopsy? That word is a heavy, vibrating question mark. It is a word that hangs in the air between doctor and patient, thick with the tension of the unknown.

We need to do a biopsy is more than a medical directive. It is a pivot point that can turn a patient's world upside down in an instant, marking the exact threshold where uncertainty meets the search for the absolute truth.

For the patient sitting on the crinkly paper of an exam table, a biopsy may be perceived as the start of a problem, a source of anxiety, a needle, a procedure, a period of agonizing waiting.

But in reality, a biopsy is the beginning of a solution. It is the moment we stop fighting a shadow in the dark and turn on the floodlights. But to understand what is happening to your body, let us look past the fear and into the language of the word itself.

To Look at Life: The Etymology of Truth

The word biopsy comes from two Greek words bios (life) and opsis (to see). Literally translated, it means to look at life. As a pathologist, this definition is my daily reality.

When a surgeon, a dermatologist, or a primary care doctor reach a limit, when they see a suspicious feature on an X ray or feel a lump beneath the skin, they are still working from the outside of a problem. They are inferring, weighing clinical signs, imaging features, signs and symptoms.

A biopsy is different. A biopsy is the moment we stop inferring and start knowing. When it works as intended, it becomes the bridge between suspicion and truth.

The Search for Microscopic Truth

Inside the Locked Skyscraper

To solve a mystery unfolding inside a massive, locked skyscraper, every member of the team must assume a distinct role.

The diagnostic radiologist is the detective stationed across the street, standing in the rain with high-powered binoculars. Through X-rays, CT scans, and MRIs, they glimpse movement behind a frosted window on the thirteenth floor. They can tell us where the target is hiding and exactly how much space it occupies; they can trace its silhouette with astonishing precision. But the glass never opens for them. They can report the 'where' and describe the suspicious behavior, but they cannot reach through the pane to name the 'who' with certainty.

The surgeon and the interventional radiologist are the tactical lead. Equipped and deliberate, they know how to navigate the building, search its hallways, and silently open the door to that room on the fourteenth floor. They control the timing, the approach, the intervention. They own the how.

And Then There Is the Pathologist

The pathologist is the forensic scientist, waiting quietly in the lab. They receive the whole story of the scene along with a single fiber lifted from the carpet. A drop of ink scraped from a letter. A fragment small enough to miss, powerful enough to decide everything. While others watch the silhouette in the window, the pathologist alone can answer the most important question of all: The who!

A surgical team without a pathology report is a team operating in the dark, unable to discern whether the figure behind the glass is a benign visitor or a lethal intruder. It is the pathologist who translates suspicion into certainty, offering the most consequential distinction in medicine: benign or malignant.

But this work is not done in isolation; the pathologist relies heavily on the surgeon and the radiologist to provide the essential piece of the 'who'. Within this intricate symbiosis, the triad of surgeon, radiologist, and pathologist stands as a formidable arsenal against the unknown.

Why the Naked Eye Is Not Enough

People often ask why a surgeon, after years of elite training and having seen thousands of organs, cannot simply look at a tumor and know its nature.

The answer lies in the deceptive camouflage of biology.

To the naked eye, a high-grade, aggressive cancer can look identical to a harmless pocket of inflamed tissue. Both may appear as firm, gray-white masses. Both can feel heavy in the hand. Both can push and distort the healthy organs around them. The eye, powerful as it is, remains a macro-tool struggling to interpret a micro-world.

Where the Truth Actually Lives

The truth of disease does not reside in the visible lump. It lives deeper. It hides in the warped architecture of cells, in the misshapen nucleus that no longer follows the rules, in the collapse of social distancing between neighboring cells, and in the way they begin to chew through the surrounding scaffolding, ignoring boundaries and rewriting order.

This is why the biopsy remains the Gold Standard. Physical exams and imaging studies are invaluable clues, strong circumstantial evidence in a complex case. But the biopsy is the microscopic evidence down to the cellular level. It is what closes the investigation. It is what turns suspicion into certainty. Only when the cells and the tissue speak under the microscope does the mystery finally reveal its identity.

The Human Behind the Glass

In the high-precision world of the laboratory, it is easy to see only the science. But I tell my team the same thing every day: behind every slide, there is someone immensely important. That sliver of tissue isn't just a specimen; it is part of a human being. It is a mother, a father, or a child who is currently holding their breath, anxiously awaiting the word that will potentially define their future.

The Hidden Doctor

One of the strangest aspects of my profession is that the pathologist is often one of the most important doctors a patient will never physically meet.

When you go to the hospital for a biopsy, you see the nurse who preps you, the specialist who performs the procedure, and the receptionist who checks you in and out. But after you leave, your tissue begins a journey into a hidden world. It goes to the pathologist.

While your primary doctor treats you, the pathologist is the one who defines what is being treated. So, as some rightfully put it, the pathologist is the doctor's doctor, providing the map that the rest of the medical team will follow.

The Three Pillars of Diagnosis

To understand why your doctor ordered a biopsy, you must understand the three ways we see disease:

Signs and Symptoms: What you feel (pain, fatigue, a lump).

Imaging: What see-through machines see (shadows, spots, densities).

Tissue Diagnosis (The Biopsy): What the cells actually are and what they tell us.

You can have the first two without the third, but you can rarely have a definitive diagnosis without the biopsy. It is the definitive word in modern medicine.

In the chapters that follow, I am going to take you behind the curtain of the laboratory

But first, let's review a quick history!

Chapter 2

A Short History of Biopsies

To see a World in a Grain of Sand, And a Heaven in a Wildflower. Hold Infinity in the palm of your hand, And Eternity in an hour.

, *William Blake*

The Era of Shadows: Medicine Before the Lens

For thousands of years, the human body was a black box. Ancient physicians in Egypt, Greece, China, India etc. were masters of observation, but their observations were limited to what the naked eye could see.

They could see a tumor growing on a neck; they could feel the heat of an infection; but they had no way of knowing what was happening inside those swollen tissues.

In this era, disease was often attributed to humors, bad air (miasma), or divine will. The idea that a disease could be identified by examining a small piece of flesh was non-existent.

Surgery was a desperate last resort, usually involving the amputation of limbs or the lancing of boils. To cut into the body just to look was considered both dangerous and sacrilegious.

The biopsy, the act of looking at life, remained impossible because we lacked the two things that define modern pathology: The Tool (The Microscope) and The Language (Cell Theory).

The First Glimmer: The 17th Century Revolution

The history of the biopsy did NOT begin with a doctor, but with a fabric merchant in Holland named Antonie van Leeuwenhoek. He wasn't looking for cancer. He was looking for the quality of threads in his shop. To do this, he created small but high-powered magnifying lenses.

When he turned those lenses away from cloth and toward a drop of pond water, and eventually his own blood, he became the first human being to see animalcules (meaning, little animals) and blood cells.

However, the medical establishment was slow to change. Even as the 1700s progressed, doctors were still macroscopic. They performed autopsies (looking at the dead) to understand the living, but they were looking at whole organs. They could say, The liver is hard, but they couldn't tell you why the liver had turned to stone.

The Birth of the Gold Standard: Rudolf Virchow

The most pivotal moment in the history of the biopsy occurred in the mid-19th century, led by a man born in Schivelbein, in the Kingdom of Prussia (modern-day Świdwin, Poland). Often called the 'Father of Modern Pathology,' Rudolf Virchow revolutionized the field while practicing in Berlin, Germany.

Before Virchow, people believed that diseases originated in organs or tissues as a whole. Virchow proposed a radical new idea: Omnis cellula e cellula (Every cell comes from a cell). He argued that disease does not start in the liver; it starts in a single cell within the liver that has gone rogue.

This was the Big Bang of pathology. If disease starts in the cell, then the only way to truly diagnose a patient is to find those cells while the patient is still alive. The shift from autopsy (seeing the dead) to biopsy (seeing the living) had begun.

The Problem of Mush: How We Learned to Slice Life

Before the mid-19th century, pathologists faced a frustrating physical barrier: human tissue is soft, wet, and mushy. If you try to slice a piece of fresh liver thin enough for light to pass through it, it simply crumbles. Because of this, pathology was largely limited to examining whole organs in jars; the fine architecture of the cell remained a blurry mystery.

1869: The Paraffin Breakthrough

The first major leap came from Swiss-German pathologist Edwin Klebs. In 1869, he introduced the revolutionary idea of supporting dehydrated tissue by saturating it in melted paraffin wax. Think of a moist piece of sponge, except instead of being soaked in water, it is fully saturated with liquid wax. As the wax cools to room temperature, it hardens, becoming as solid as a candle. This process produces a firm, stable block that can be sliced into thin, translucent sections, a feat earlier wet preservation methods could never achieve.

This breakthrough transformed pathology from a fragile, imprecise practice into a reliable science. For the first time, tissue architecture could be preserved permanently and examined repeatedly. What had once been soft, distorted material became a stable, transparent record, laying the foundation for modern diagnostic pathology.

The 1880s: Refining the Craft

By the early 1880s, these methods were refined into a sophisticated science. Histologist Wilhelm His Sr. improved the process by first dehydrating tissue in alcohol and clearing it in essential oils, such as lavender, before applying the molten wax. This allowed the paraffin to fully permeate the cells, making the tissue much more reliable to cut. During this same era, pioneers like Victor von Ebner helped shape the foundations of modern microscopic anatomy, perfecting the chemistry required to see the invisible.

The 1880s: The Microtome (The Ultimate Deli Slicer)

To take advantage of these new wax blocks, engineers perfected the microtome. Think of this as the world's most precise deli slicer. It allowed histotechs to shave off sections of tissue so incredibly thin, often only 4 to 5 microns, that they were only one cell layer thick. To put it in perspective, it's so thin that about seventeen of these slices would equal the thickness of a single human hair (See figure 4-1 in Chapter 4).

1893: Formalin (The Time-Freezer)

The moment biological tissue is disconnected from its blood supply, it enters a state of immediate crisis; enzymes begin to consume cells from the inside out, initiating the inevitable chemistry of decay. Historically, this meant that the intricate architecture of life would vanish within hours, leaving little for science to observe. However, the final piece of the puzzle fell into place in 1893 when Ferdinand Blum discovered that formaldehyde (formalin) possessed a remarkable power to arrest this dissolution.

By fixing the body's proteins, formalin binds molecules together and silences the enzymatic reactions that drive decomposition. This chemical intervention essentially freezes time, transforming fleeting, living matter into a durable, permanent record. Because formalin holds the shape and relationships of cells fast, it allowed biology to be paused for the first time in history, providing generations of observers the opportunity to study the frozen architecture of life long after it would have otherwise slipped away.

The Result: A Library of Human Life

The durability of these paraffin-embedded specimens became their greatest strength. Because these blocks are stable at room temperature, they create a permanent biological archive. Modern reviews affirm that these samples can remain intact for generations.

In archives held by some of the oldest pathology institutions in the United States and across Europe, wax-encased tissue blocks have endured for well over a century. Preserved in paraffin, these specimens remain stable at room temperature for decades and often far longer, forming vast historical collections that continue to be used worldwide.

Because these samples can still be retrieved today, they allow us to reopen a patient's story with tools that were unimaginable to the scientists who first prepared them. Modern genetic sequencing and molecular analysis can illuminate details that 19th-century pioneers could never have foreseen.

What once would have seemed like science fiction is now routine practice, proof that these humble wax blocks are not just relics of medical history, but living archives that continue to teach, diagnose, and reveal.

The First Living Diagnosis: Frozen-Section

In the late nineteenth and early twentieth centuries, a transformative technique known as the frozen section emerged. Surgeons at leading institutions, including Johns Hopkins, realized that tissue could be removed while a patient was still on the operating table, rapidly frozen using carbon dioxide, and examined under a microscope within minutes. For the first time, pathology could inform surgical decisions in real time.

The stakes were extraordinary. The patient lay anesthetized; the surgeon paused, scalpel in hand; and the pathologist had only minutes to answer a defining question: Is this cancer? Or Are the margins clear? The response would determine the extent of surgery, whether to remove an entire breast or preserve as much tissue as possible. In these moments, the pathologist assumed a quiet but commanding role, guiding the course of the operation with authority born of microscopic evidence.

That legacy endures today. Pathology remains an essential partner in surgery, with frozen-section services integrated into operating rooms at virtually every hospital worldwide. Although the technology has advanced, from carbon dioxide to liquid nitrogen and precision cryostats, the urgency has not changed. Surgeons still pause mid-procedure, relying on pathologists to deliver immediate, high-confidence diagnoses. In this way, frozen-section pathology continues to serve as surgery's real-time compass, steering clinical decisions with clarity drawn from the cellular level.

The Evolution of Tissue Processing: From Patience to Pressure

Before the advent of automated tissue processors, histology was a discipline defined by patience, timing, and hands-on skill. Once the specimen had been examined by eye, the histotechnician became the steward of its journey, guiding the tissue through a carefully choreographed sequence of dehydration, clearing, and wax infiltration.

Water was removed gradually through successive alcohol baths of increasing strength, a process that demanded hours of close attention to ensure the tissue was properly prepared. The specimen was then transferred to xylene, which replaced the alcohol and rendered the tissue translucent, a critical and delicate transition before embedding.

From there, the tissue entered molten paraffin wax inside a heated oven. In a practice that favored gentleness over speed, technicians often allowed the wax to infiltrate slowly overnight as the oven cooled, preserving even the most fragile cellular structures. The following morning, the specimen was given a final immersion in fresh wax before the technician completed the art of embedding.

This slow, deliberate method has largely been replaced by modern automation, but it stands as a reminder that early histology was not merely a process but a well-practiced craft.

While this traditional method took a full 24 to 48 hours from start to finish, modern fluid-transfer processors now use vacuum pressure and heat to achieve the same results in as little as 4 - 8 hours.

The Dark Age of Stigma (1920s - 1950s)

Strangely, as the technology improved, a new obstacle emerged: Fear. During the mid-20th century, a common myth took hold. People (and even some doctors) believed that sticking a needle into a tumor would disturb the cancer and cause it to spread throughout the body. Because of this, many biopsies were delayed until it was too late.

It took decades of rigorous clinical trials to prove that a biopsy is a safe, life-saving necessity. The transition from the fear of the needle to the necessity of the needle defines the mid-century evolution of pathology.

The Modern Frontier: Beyond the Visible

As we moved into the 1980s and 1990s, the history of the biopsy took another leap. We moved from Looking at the Shape to Looking at the Signature.

We developed Immunohistochemistry (IHC). These are special designer stains that act like heat-seeking missiles. They only stick to specific proteins. This allowed pathologists to say, Not only is this cancer, but it is a cancer that started in the lung some time ago and has now moved to the bone.

2026 and Beyond: The Digital Rebirth

Today, we are living in the most exciting chapter of this history. We are moving from glass to gigabytes.

During my residency at Hahnemann, we handled only glass slides for diagnostic work. Today, we can scan those slides into high-definition digital images that we call whole slide imaging or in short WSI.

We are also seeing the rise of the Liquid Biopsy, finding fragments of cancer DNA in a simple tube of blood. While this hasn't replaced the tissue biopsy (the gold standard), it represents the next step in our ancient quest: to see the invisible without ever needing a scalpel.

Why History Matters to You

I tell this story because every time a patient has a biopsy today, they are benefiting from centuries of accidents, genius, and persistence. When you look at that tiny specimen container, you aren't just looking at a piece of tissue. You are looking at the culmination of Van Leeuwenhoek's lenses, Virchow's theories, and the chemistry of a thousand labs. We have moved from the shadows to the light and in doing so, we have given millions of people a chance at a second chapter in their lives.

The Martyrdom of the Early Pathologists

History books often paint the evolution of science as a series of clean, intellectual breakthroughs. In reality, the history of pathology was written in blood. Before we understood germ theory or the importance of PPE (Personal Protective Equipment), the pathology lab was one of the most dangerous places to work.

In the 19th century, pathologists like Rudolf Virchow and his contemporaries were performing autopsies and examining biopsies of patients with tuberculosis, syphilis, and streptococcal infections with their bare hands.

A single nick of the finger from a scalpel or a needle could be a death sentence. We have records of dozens of young physicians who died of prosector's paronychia, a polite Victorian term for overwhelming sepsis contracted from a patient's tissue.

These early pioneers were the first to realize that tissue wasn't just a map; it was a biological record that remained active even after it left the body. Their sacrifices led to the invention of rubber gloves, the use of antiseptic fixatives like formalin, and the rigorous safety protocols we use in 2026.

Every time a modern lab technician safely handles a specimen, they are standing on the shoulders of those who paid for our safety with their lives.

The Evolution of the Needle: From Harpoon to Whisper

If the microscope is the eye of pathology, the biopsy needle is its hand. The history of how we physically get the tissue out of the body is a story of moving from the macro to the micro.

In the early days, a biopsy usually meant a surgeon cutting a large, painful wedge of tissue out of a patient while they were awake or lightly sedated. It was a traumatic event.

By the 1930s, doctors in New York and Sweden began experimenting with Fine Needle Aspiration (FNA). They realized that if you used a needle, you could suck out enough cells to make a diagnosis without ever needing a stitch.

This was revolutionary, but it faced massive pushback. Traditionalists argued that a few cells weren't enough to see the architecture of the disease. They were right, in a way, which led to the invention of the Core Needle.

The Core Needle is a masterpiece of engineering. It's a hollow tube with a guillotine mechanism inside that captures a perfect cylinder of tissue, a little thicker than a pencil lead.

Today, we have vacuum-assisted needles that can take multiple samples through a single tiny hole. We have gone from harpooning the disease to whispering to it, taking only what we need with surgical precision and minimal recovery time for the patient.

The Architect's Final Plan

We have traveled from the Animalcules of the 1600s to the WSI of the 2020s. We have moved from seeing the body as a collection of humors to seeing it as a digital code that can be cracked.

The history books close here. From the next chapter forward, we step into the pathology laboratory as it works today — and you will see why the part of a biopsy that frightens patients most is often the part that should give them the most hope.

Chapter 3

The Harvest: How a Biopsy Is Taken

Knowledge is the antidote to fear.

Ralph Waldo Emerson

The Surgical Strike

In my years as a medical student and then as a general practitioner, I learned that the most important part of any procedure happens before the first incision is made. It is the moment of mental preparation, the realization that you are about to breach the body's most sacred boundary: the skin.

A biopsy is often described as a minor procedure. But for the person on the table, there is nothing minor about it. Whether it is a tiny punch of the skin or a core needle into the breast, a biopsy is a surgical strike. It is the moment when all the consultation and a definitive intervention begins.

In this chapter, we will walk through the how and why of these procedures, breaking down the wall of mystery that surrounds the specimen container.

The Tool for the Task: Why Techniques Differ

One of the most common questions patients ask is, Why can't you just use a needle for everything? To understand the answer, you have to think of the human body not as a single mass, but as a complex landscape of different textures.

Biopsy Types by Collection Methods

- **Fine Needle Aspiration (FNA):** A thin needle removes cell clusters.
- **Core Needle Biopsy:** removes a core cylinder of solid tissue.
- **Incisional Biopsy:** removes a small piece of a mass.
- **Excisional Biopsy:** The entire lesion is removed.

A lung is like a sponge; a liver is like firm pâté; a bone is like a piece of oak; and the skin is like a multi-layered suit of armor. You cannot use a sponge-tool to sample an oak tree. Consequently, we have developed a specialized arsenal for the harvest.

1. The Skin Punch and Shave

The skin is the most frequently biopsied organ. Because it is our external shield, we can access it easily.

The Shave: Think of this like a very precise carpenter's plane. The doctor/provider uses a small blade to take a thin shaving of the top layers. This is ideal for superficial growths.

The Punch: This is my favorite tool for its simplicity. It looks like a tiny, circular cookie cutter. With a quick twizzle of the fingers, it takes a perfect cylinder of skin, reaching down into the fatty layers where sometimes deeper diseases hide.

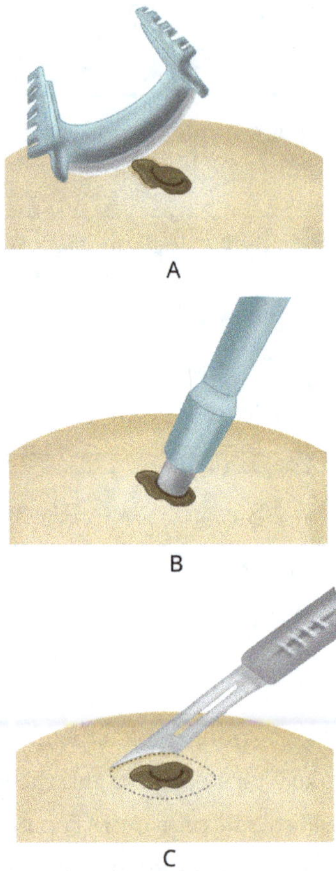

Figure 1. A. Shave biopsy; B: Puch biopsy; C: Excisional biopsy

2. The Fine Needle Aspiration (FNA)

This is the whisper of the biopsy world. Using a needle thinner than the one used for your annual blood draw, the doctor moves the needle back and forth within a lump (usually in the thyroid or a lymph node). This doesn't take a chunk of tissue; it sucks out a few thousand individual cells.

When possible, aspiration fluid can be taken for making a cell block.

A cell block is prepared by concentrating aspiration fluid via centrifugation, which causes the suspended cells and tissue fragments to sediment into a cohesive pellet. This pellet is then processed and embedded in paraffin, allowing for thin-sectioning and a comprehensive histological evaluation similar to a traditional tissue biopsy.

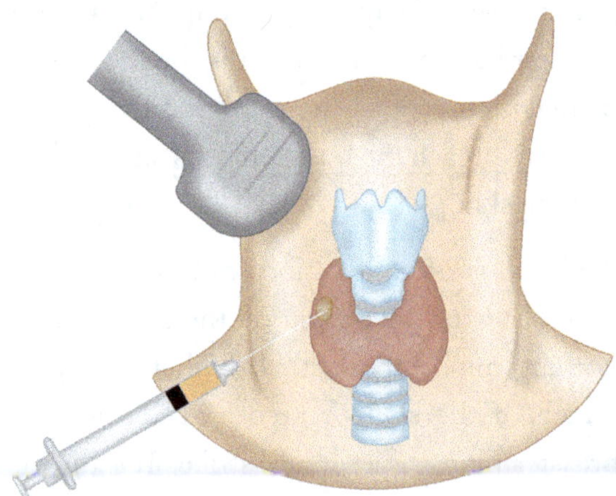

Figure 2. Ultrasound guided thyroid fine needle aspiration biopsy

3. The Core Needle

If the FNA is a whisper, the Core Needle is a clear, louder statement. This needle is hollow and spring-loaded. When the provider fires the needle, it captures a solid core of tissue. This is the gold standard for breast and prostate biopsies because the pathologist needs to see the architecture, how the cells are arranged next to each other, not just the cells themselves.

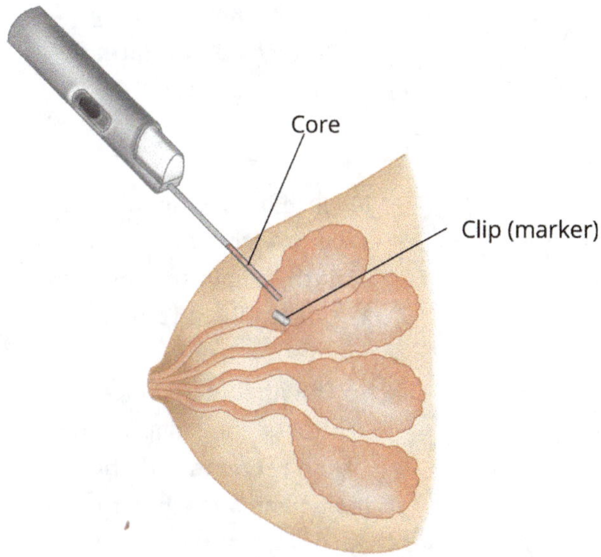

Figure 3. Core needle biopsy

The Journey into the Deep: Imaging-Guided Biopsies

What happens when the lump is deep inside the body, tucked behind the ribs or nestled near the spine? In the old days, this required an Open Biopsy, a full surgery under general anesthesia just to get a sample. Today, we use GPS for the Body. Interventional Radiology (IR). Using a live CT scan or an Ultrasound, the doctor can watch the needle move through the body in real-time. On the screen, they see the needle tip inching toward the target. They can avoid major blood vessels and nerves with millimeter precision. This has turned what used to be a hospital stay into a 45-minute outpatient appointment.

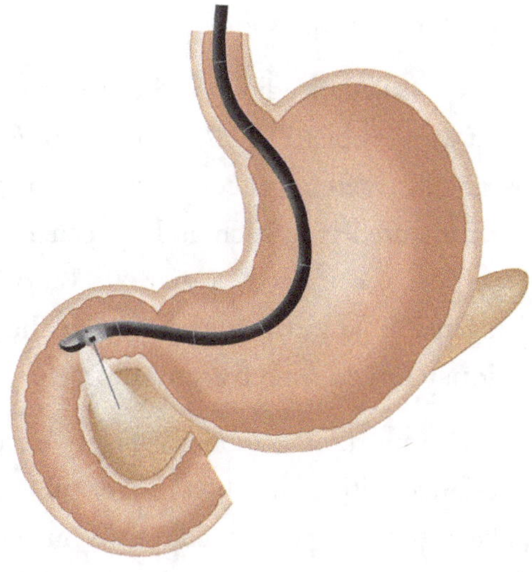

Figure 4. Endoscopic ultrasound guided biopsy of the pancreas. An example of imaging guided biopsy.

The Specimen Container: The Holy Grail of the Lab

Once the tissue is harvested, it is placed into a small plastic cup filled with formalin (usually) or other preservative fluid. Most patients never think twice about this container, but for a pathologist, this is where the Chain of Custody begins.

Those steps — what happens to the specimen container after it leaves the operating room — are the subject of the next chapter.

Debunking the Great Myth: Does a Biopsy Spread Cancer?

As I briefly mentioned in previous chapter, in every country I have practiced, from Ethiopia to Canada and the United States, I have heard the same terrifying whisper: *'If you poke a cancer, it spreads'.* Even as recently as three months ago, a physician from outside the USA has asked me this question.

This is called 'Seeding,' and I want to be as direct as possible: For 99.9% of biopsies, this is a myth. Even in cancers with a slightly higher documented risk, such as liver cancer (HCC), the rate of seeding is a mere 0.1% to 0.7%, **a negligible shadow compared to the light a biopsy sheds on a treatment path**.

Most importantly, modern biopsy needles are designed with a sheath, an outer tube that acts like a tunnel. The needle goes in, takes the sample, and is pulled back inside the sheath before it ever leaves the body. The captured cancer cells never touch the healthy tissue on the way out.

Furthermore, thousands of medical studies have compared patients who had biopsies to those who didn't. There is no evidence that a biopsy changes the stage of a cancer or makes it travel faster. In fact, the only thing that spreads cancer is waiting too long to find out what it is. A biopsy is the tool we use to stop a spread, not start it.

Author Tip: Why Biopsies Don't Spread Cancer

Modern biopsy needles are built with a **protective sheath**—an outer tube that acts like a tunnel.

The needle advances, collects the sample, and then **retracts fully back inside the sheath before it exits.**

Any captured cells remain **contained within the needle system,** so they don't touch healthy tissue on the way out.

This design makes modern biopsies both **precise and safe.**

The Patient's Experience: What to Expect

If you are reading this because you are scheduled for a biopsy, here is the insider's view of what you will experience:

The Numbing: The most noticeable sensation is usually the local anesthetic. You may feel a brief pinch or warmth that lasts just a few seconds. Once the area is numb, you should feel pressure, but not sharp pain.

The Click: If a Core Needle is being used, you will hear a loud click or pop, much like a heavy-duty stapler. This is the spring-loaded mechanism taking the sample. It may be startling, but it is fast.

The Pressure: After the procedure, the nurse will hold firm pressure on the site for several minutes. Since we aren't using large stitches, we rely on the body's natural clotting to seal the tiny needle track.

The Sample Adequacy: Why We Take Multiple Pieces in Core Biopsies

You might notice the doctor taking three, four, or even six cores from the same lesion. This is because of tumor heterogeneity.

A tumor is not a uniform block of cells/tissue. It is a neighborhood, if you may. Some parts of it might be quiet (benign), while other parts are rioting (cancerous). By taking multiple samples, the clinician ensures that the pathologist gets a representative view of the entire area. Much like seeing the whole city represented, not just one street corner.

Our goal is to give you a definitive answer the first time, so you receive the right treatment immediately and, most importantly, so you never have to return for a repeat biopsy because the first sample was 'non-representative'.

The Pathology Hand-Off

As the procedure ends and the final bandage is placed, the harvest is complete and the journey begins. The clinician places the sample in a sealed container, which is then sent to the pathology laboratory as part of the facility's normal specimen transport process.

Inside, suspended in clear formalin, is tissue that only moments ago was part of your living body. In that instant, it undergoes a quiet transformation. It is no longer muscle or skin or gland. It becomes evidence. A message. A question waiting to be answered.

You leave the clinic and go home to rest. The discomfort fades, the day resumes, and life continues. But the cells you left behind are just beginning their work.

The Gift of the Sample

A biopsy is, at its core, a gift of information. It is a courageous act by the patient and an act of precision by the clinician. By allowing a small piece of your body to be sampled, you offer your medical team the one thing no scan or symptom can fully provide: certainty. You hand them the key to a locked door.

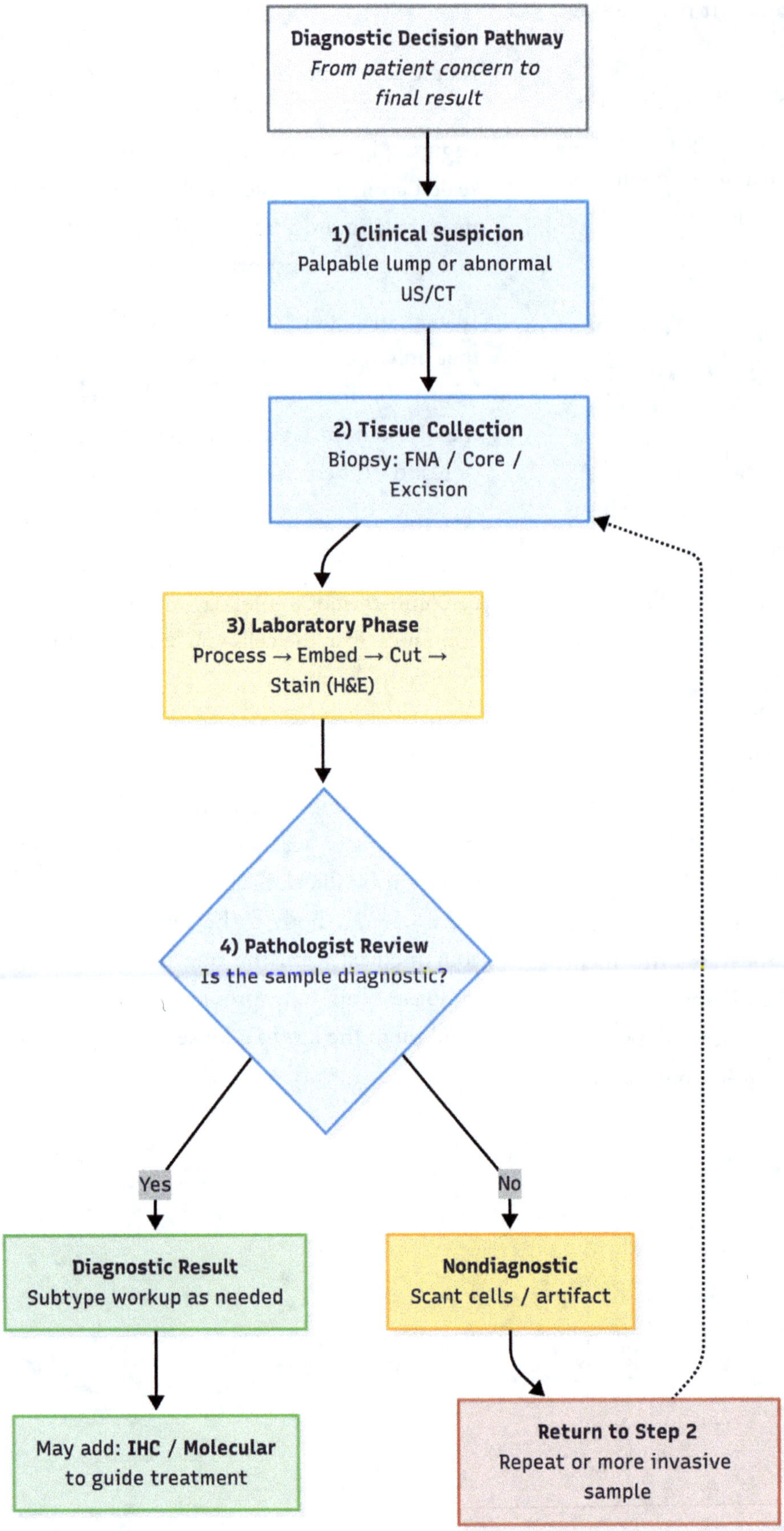
Diagnostic Decision Pathway
From patient concern to final result
1) Clinical Suspicion
Palpable lump or abnormal US/CT
2) Tissue Collection
Biopsy: FNA / Core / Excision
3) Laboratory Phase
Process → Embed → Cut → Stain (H&E)
4) Pathologist Review
Is the sample diagnostic?
Yes
No
Diagnostic Result
Subtype workup as needed
May add: **IHC / Molecular** to guide treatment
Nondiagnostic
Scant cells / artifact
Return to Step 2
Repeat or more invasive sample

Chapter 4

From Clinic to Lab: The Journey of Your Tissue

The biopsy is the most honest conversation your body will ever have with your doctor.

The Secret City: A Backstage Pass to the Pathology Laboratory

If a hospital were a bustling city, the Pathology Laboratory would be its quiet intelligence headquarters, out of sight, highly secure, and essential to every important decision. It is a world of white coats, softly humming machines, and an unwavering focus on accuracy.

The journey between the biopsy procedure room and the microscope is a carefully choreographed process. We're going to follow your tissue through the Secret City of the pathology lab, where a tiny piece of your tissue is transformed into a permanent, microscopic record, one that helps guide life-changing medical decisions.

Step 1: Accessioning, The Chain of Custody

The most critical moment for a biopsy isn't always the procedure itself, it's the hand-off.

In a large hospital, thousands of specimens move through the system every day: a skin sample from dermatology, a lung biopsy from the floors, a gallbladder from surgery. Each one represents a real person, waiting for answers.

The first stop is the Accessioning sub-department of the lab, the laboratory's version of patient admissions. Every container is carefully matched to the doctor's order. Names, birthdates, and specimen details are verified. If the lab is equipped with the technology, a unique barcode is created, and from that moment forward, your tissue is digitally tracked at every step.

If even a single letter does not match, everything stops. In any patient care environment including the laboratory, there is no such thing as close enough. Any labeling discrepancy is treated with the highest level of seriousness, because accuracy at this step avoids mismatches and protects patients.

Errors involving specimen mismatches do occur in medicine. When they happen, they most often arise during specimen collection and handoff, not within the laboratory itself. That distinction matters. Modern pathology laboratories apply extraordinarily strict accessioning procedures, and once a specimen is accessioned, it is tracked with redundant identifiers and digital barcodes that are designed to be nearly foolproof.

As a laboratory director, I allow no margin for error at this stage, or at any other point in the specimen processing cycle. Precision here is not a preference. It is a responsibility and a matter of patient safety.

Step 2: The Gross Room, Seeing the Big Picture

Next, the specimen enters the Gross Room. The word gross doesn't mean unpleasant, it comes from the German groß, meaning large or overall. This is where the first hands-on examination happens. In the regulatory legal terminology, it is a high complexity testing.

The specimen is carefully described in detail: its size, color, texture, and shape. If the tissue came from a larger mass or tumor, something especially important happens here, we create a map.

The outer surface of the tissue is painted with different colored inks to mark its original orientation in the body. Blue might represent the top, like the sky; green might mark the bottom, like the earth. These colors create a map, allowing us to know exactly where each part of the specimen came from in relation to the patient's anatomy.

Even after the tissue is sliced into thin microscopic sections, the ink remains visible. Under the microscope, those colors tell us precisely which edge of the specimen we're looking at. Because of this, we can report to the surgeon not only whether a surgical margin is positive, but exactly where on the patient's body that margin corresponds to, and where additional treatment or re-excision may be necessary.

Once the key areas are identified, small representative samples are placed into a labeled plastic rectangular fenestrated box we call a cassette, a protective holder that carries the tissue through the next stages.

Step 3: Fixation, Freezing Time

As we discussed in the previous chapter, once tissue is harvested and placed into the specimen container, the Chain of Custody begins. The 10% Neutral Buffered Formalin inside that container is there to stop the clock.

When it comes to this chemical freezing, timing is everything. We look for a Goldilocks window to ensure the record remains permanent and readable:

Too little time: The formalin doesn't fully penetrate the tissue, leaving it vulnerable for decay and making a diagnosis challenging.

Too much time: The chemical bonds can become too crowded, damaging delicate DNA and making advanced molecular testing, much harder.

The general rule of thumb to ensure the specimen is properly preserved, is to immerse the specimen inside a formalin container with at least 10 times more volume than the specimen itself.

During this window, the tissue's structure is locked into place. It is a chemical preservation that captures the cells exactly as they were, mid-story. By halting the decay, we transform a fading biological sample into a pristine, permanent record that allows us to see the truth of the biopsy under the microscope.

Step 4: Processing, The Great Exchange

To examine tissue under a microscope, it must be sliced thinner than a human hair. But tissue is mostly water, and water is soft. To make it firm enough to slice, as mentioned in chapter 2, we replace the water with wax.

This happens overnight in an automated processor through a precise series of steps:

- Dehydration: Alcohol removes all water
- Clearing: A special solution removes the alcohol
- Infiltration: Warm liquid paraffin wax fills every microscopic space

By morning, the tissue is no longer flimsy, it's supported from within.

Step 5: Embedding, Creating the Master File

The tissue is carefully positioned in a small mold, and additional liquid wax is poured around it. As the wax cools, it solidifies into a smooth white block. This block becomes the permanent record, the master file, and can be safely stored. If the pathologist needs further stains after the initial microscopic review, new slides can be cut from this same master block.

Should new questions arise long after the original diagnosis, the very same block can be retrieved and examined again using technologies that may not even exist today. It is a biological time capsule, preserving the tissue exactly as it was on the day it was taken.

However, each time thin sections are cut, the block becomes slightly smaller. Over many recuts, the tissue can eventually be depleted. When that point is reached, the block is considered exhausted, and no further slides can be made.

Step 6: Microtomy, The Ultimate Slice

Now comes one of the most delicate steps of all. The wax block is mounted onto a microtome. Each slice is only about 4-5 microns thick. For comparison, a human hair is about 70 microns thick.

The slices form a ribbon so delicate that even a breath of air could disturb it. These sections are gently floated on warm water bath to smooth them, then carefully lifted onto glass slides.

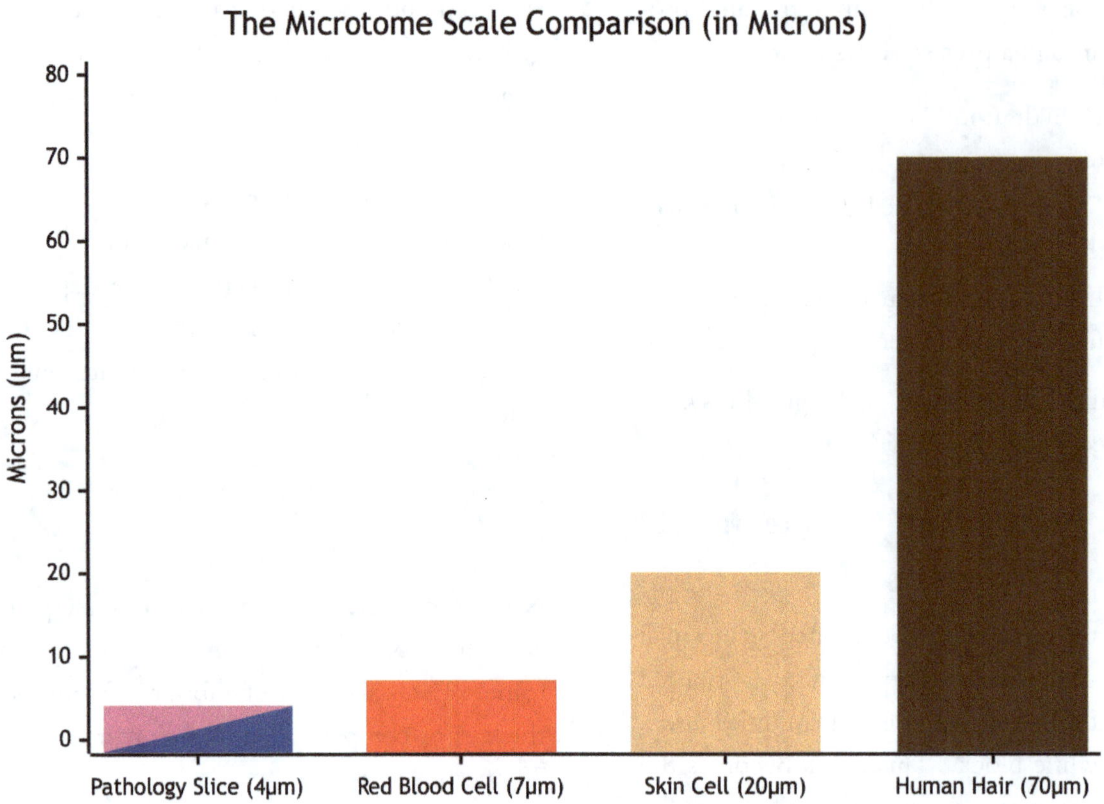

Figure 4-1 Illustration showing thickness comparison at the microtome scale.

Step 7: Staining, Revealing the Pink and Blue World

At this stage, the tissue is nearly invisible. To reveal its structure, it must be stained. The slides travel through an automated stainer, most importantly through two dyes: Hematoxylin (blue-purple): highlights the nucleus, the cell's control center. Eosin (pink): highlights the surrounding cell body and tissues. A thin glass coverslip is sealed on top. The journey is complete. A slide is now ready be examined under the microscope.

What I am actually looking for at the microscope — and how the art and science of microscopic examination turns these glass slides into answers — is the subject of the next chapter.

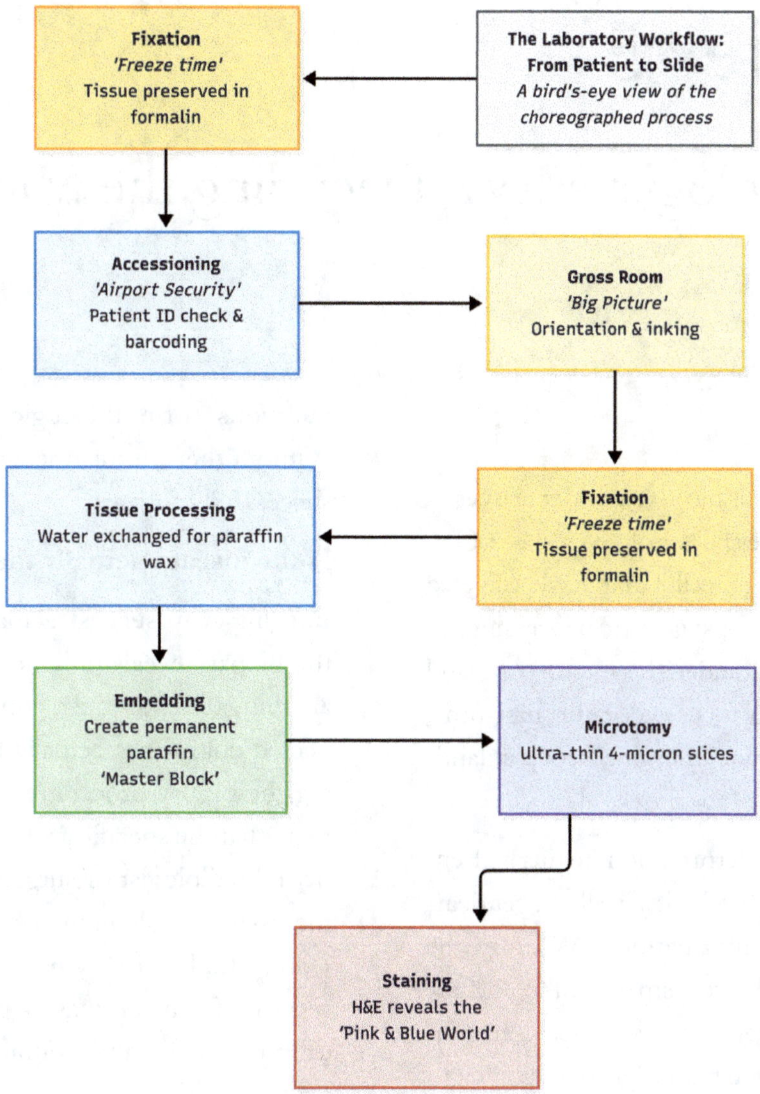
The Laboratory Workflow: From Patient to Slide
A bird's-eye view of the choreographed process
Fixation
'Freeze time'
Tissue preserved in formalin
Accessioning
'Airport Security'
Patient ID check & barcoding
Gross Room
'Big Picture'
Orientation & inking
Fixation
'Freeze time'
Tissue preserved in formalin
Tissue Processing
Water exchanged for paraffin wax
Embedding
Create permanent paraffin 'Master Block'
Microtomy
Ultra-thin 4-micron slices
Staining
H&E reveals the 'Pink & Blue World'

Chapter 5

The Pathologist's Eye: Decoding the Microscopic Landscape

The Moment of Focus

A few days after your biopsy, a folder arrives at my desk. Inside are slides holding a slice of tissue with millions of cells that have traveled through the different stages of processing. I place the first slide under the microscope and gently bring it into focus. For the first time, human eyes examine the microscopic landscape of your biopsy specimen.

This is where my interpretation begins as I enter a world that is paradoxically silent, yet deafeningly loud with information. As I turn the focus knob, the blurred smears of colorfully stained cells sharpen, one as intricate and intentional as a satellite map of a sprawling city.

In this chapter, we explore how pathologists are trained to look beyond the surface, how they study the ways your cells communicate, how those cells construct their surrounding architecture, and ultimately, what their growth patterns reveal about their true intentions and identity.

The Initial Three Fundamental Questions

Every time I sit down at my microscope and bring a slide into focus, I am searching for answers to three fundamental questions. These questions form the logic gate of medicine. Without them, a treatment plan may not move successfully forward.

Is the disease actually there?

Imaging may suggest a mass, but sometimes the biopsy reveals only normal tissue. Before anything else, I must confirm that the suspected culprit has actually been captured during the biopsy procedure. This involves verifying that the specific area of concern identified by the radiologist or surgeon is present within the tissue sample I am viewing on the slide. If I don't find it, I may have to order additional sections from the master paraffin block. We call this deeper level examination.

If the biopsy reveals abnormality, then what exactly is it?

Medicine has moved far beyond the binary of cancer or not cancer. Is the process slow-growing or aggressive? My role is to name the disease accurately, ensuring my observation matches the clinical findings. I must identify the specific subtype of the disease and, if applicable, its grade, to determine how the cells are likely to behave and respond to treatment protocols.

If we're looking at a cancerous growth, where does it end?

When surgeons remove a tumor, I examine the edges (margins). If abnormal cells extend to the border, the disease remains. I provide a measurement of the distance between the abnormal cells and the outer edge of the tissue to help the surgeon decide if further surgery is required to achieve clear boundaries.

The Power of Perspective: Low to High

A diagnosis is not made at a single magnification. It is a process of zooming in and out, much like an investigator at a crime scene.

The 2x and 4x View: The Bird's Eye (Architecture)

I always start at the lowest magnification (2x or 4x). This is the scanning phase. At this level, I cannot see individual cells clearly; instead, I see the architecture.

Healthy tissue is organized. It has zoning laws. In a liver, the cells should form neat plates. In a colon, they should form orderly glands that look like a row of test tubes.

When I see a disturbance in the force, a place where the neat rows have been replaced by a chaotic jumble, that is my first red flag. Abnormality, at its core, is a loss of architectural discipline.

The 10x View

Once I find a suspicious area, I zoom in. Now I am looking at how the cells interact with their neighbors.

Invasion: This is the most critical word in my vocabulary. Healthy cells stay within their boundaries (the property line). Cancer cells are trespassers.

In healthy tissue, cells follow a rigorous architectural plan; they are 'social' and organized. When I look through the lens, I am looking for a breakdown in that order. I look for 'atypical' nuclei, cells whose command centers have become enlarged, dark, and irregular.

I look for a loss of polarity, where cells forget which way is up and begin to pile onto one another in a chaotic, crowded heap. It is this transition from a disciplined community to a lawless crowd that reveals the presence of disease.

Inflammation: Sometimes the chaos isn't cancer; it's a war. I look for the police of the body, e.g. lymphocytes, histiocytes, neutrophils. If the area is flooded with tiny, dark purple dots (white blood cells), I know I'm looking at an infection or an autoimmune battle.

The 20x and 40x View: The Individual (The Face of the Cell)

Finally, I go to high power. This is where I look at the individual cell. I am specifically looking at the nucleus and the cytoplasm of the cells.

The Size: A cancer cell nucleus takes up more space than it should.

The Chromatin: I look at the DNA coil inside the nucleus. In a healthy cell, it's fine and light. In a cancer cell, it looks like clumpy coal.

Mitosis: I look for cells in the act of dividing. In a healthy adult, cells divide slowly. If I see a mitotic figure, a nucleus caught in the act of pulling itself apart, it means the tissue is growing rapidly. If I see lots of them, possibly I am looking at a high-grade tumor.

The Art of the Differential Diagnosis

My mind works like a biological search engine. Every pattern I see triggers a list of possibilities called a Differential Diagnosis.

Imagine I see a cluster of clear, pale cells in a kidney biopsy.

1. Could it be Clear Cell Renal Cell Carcinoma (a common cancer)?
2. Could it be Xanthogranulomatous Pyelonephritis (a rare infection)?
3. Could it be a normal variation of the tissue?

To narrow this down, I may use Special Stains or immunohistochemical stains. For example, if the cells turn brown for a protein called PAX8, I know for certain they are kidney cells.

Navigating the Gray Zones, The Honesty of Uncertainty

Patients often expect pathology reports to deliver certainty in bold, uncomplicated terms: Benign. Malignant. Yes. No. When they instead encounter phrases that feel cautious or ambiguous, frustration is understandable.

However, biology rarely moves in a straight, predictable line from Healthy to Cancer. Instead, there is a complex and treacherous grey zone reported as dysplasia, atypia, indeterminate etc.

In this Gray Zone, cells are misbehaving. Their architecture is distorted and their growth is irregular, but they have not yet committed the ultimate biological crime of invading surrounding tissue.

They borrow features from cancer while retaining traces of normalcy. Drawing the line between the two, determining exactly when a cell has crossed the point of no return, is the most challenging aspect of my profession and the focus of my most intensive training.

When my report identifies High-grade Dysplasia or Severe Atypia, it serves as a critical clinical alarm. It communicates a clear message to the surgeon: while this is not yet a malignancy (cancer), it could be on an inevitable trajectory towards becoming one. To call these cells malignant risks overtreatment and harm; to dismiss them risks missing a window for a cure.

When uncertainty appears in a report, it is not indecision, it is honesty. It is the pathologist raising a yellow flag, signaling that the evidence has not yet crossed the threshold of certainty. This is the moment when we order additional stains, request molecular tests, or invite a second pathologist with more experience on the particular biopsy type, to review the slide. In medicine, I don't know yet can be the safest and most ethical answer a patient can receive.

When I was practicing in Canada, every morning I would arrive at my desk to find a stack of these Gray Zones waiting for me, cases sent in consultation from other pathologists. One might belong to a young woman with a changing mole, fearful that it could be melanoma. Another might come from an elderly man whose worsening rash raised concern for a possible skin lymphoma.

I am always acutely aware that a diagnosis in either direction can alter a patient's life forever. The responsibility is immense. When the answer finally comes, it must be the right one. The weight of that truth, of knowing that the next steps in someone's life hinge on my interpretation, never leaves me.

The Pathology Report

After analyzing the slides and reviewing the special stains, my final task is to translate these visual patterns into a Pathology Report. This document is a precise fusion of scientific analysis, a legal record, and a tactical letter to the clinical team.

Precision is paramount. We utilize standardized grading systems, such as the Gleason Score for prostate cancer or the Nottingham Grade for breast cancer. These scores act as a biologic thermometer, measuring how aggressively the cells are behaving. A low-grade tumor closely resembles normal tissue and tends to grow slowly while a high-grade tumor appears as a chaotic explosion of cells, signaling a much more aggressive disease.

This report is the final destination of the harvest and the journey we have tracked in previous chapters.

The Humanity Behind the Lens

We provide precise answers so the patient can gain something essential in the fight against disease: a head start on cure.

There is a common misconception that because pathologists work in quiet rooms away from the bedside, we are detached from our patients. The reality is quite the opposite. Even in the stillness of the lab, I feel the weight of the person on the other side of the glass.

At the microscope, I scan hundreds of cells a minute, searching for the one that breaks the rules. By day's end, I may have examined millions of cells.

This work demands an intense level of focus and pattern recognition that even advanced computers still struggle to match. I am looking for the glitch in the system, the cell that has abandoned its role in the body and chosen a destructive path.

I see landscapes of colorfully stained cells on the slides from the biopsies. Yet the connection to the person behind each slide is never lost. Every specimen represents someone waiting for an answer.

I remember a case that showed just how dramatically the microscope can overturn even a confident clinical assumption.

A middle-aged patient presented with a small, firm nodule above their eyebrow, mobile, subcutaneous, and classic for an epidermal inclusion cyst. To the naked eye and the clinician's touch, it seemed routine.

Even at low power, the slide supported that impression: an inflamed cyst. It would have been easy to agree. But a subtle shift in the architecture caught my attention. I moved to high power, and the supposed inflammation vanished. What emerged instead was uniform round blue cells crashed together.

This was no benign cyst, it was Merkel cell carcinoma, an exceptionally rare and aggressive skin cancer hiding in plain sight. Under the highest magnification, the cells revealed their signature salt and pepper nuclei, the defining feature of neuroendocrine cancer. In that moment, the quiet of my office grew heavy. I was the only per-son who knew that their minor cyst was something far more dangerous.

Merkel cell carcinoma spreads with relent-less speed. Because of that microscopic discovery, they received the urgent treatment and follow-up they needed. The satisfaction of catching such a lethal disease early, and knowing it saved their life, is in-describable.

That is the profound, often unseen power of the pathologist's eye: the ability to see past the obvious and uncover the hidden threat. We provide precise answers so the patient can gain something essential in the fight against disease: a head start on cure.

Signing a pathology report is not merely completing paperwork, it is closing a chapter in a patient's story and delivering an answer to one of the most important questions they may ever ask. This is why the biopsy sits at the center of medicine: it is where the physical world of tissue meets the intellectual world of diagnosis.

By the time you finish this book, you will understand that even the smallest fragment of tissue contains a vast, intricate world, one that pathologists navigate every day with attention to its profound and often hidden depths.

From the microscope, the work moves to the page. The next chapter shows you how to read the pathology report itself — how to translate the jargon and use what you find there to advocate for your own care.

Chapter 6

Reading the Code: How to Understand Your Pathology Report

The Paper Fortress

You are sitting in your doctor's office, or perhaps you are logged into a patient portal at midnight, your heart hammering against your ribs. You open the file. You expect a clear answer: Everything is fine or Here is the problem. Instead, you are met with a wall of text that looks like it was written in a combination of Latin, Greek, and computer code.

Compound melanocytic nevus, moderately atypical, biopsy edges free of lesion Comment: Immunohistochemical stain with PRAME antibody is negative. The stain with Melan-A highlights the lesions cells.

To a patient, this feels like a fortress designed to keep you out. But this document is the most important map of the result of your biopsy. It is the finalized translation of the colorful cellular landscapes we've discussed. In this chapter, we are going to tear down that fortress. I am going to show you how to read your report like a pathologist, so you can walk into your next appointment not as a bystander, but as an informed partner in your own care.

The Anatomy of a Report

Almost every pathology report follows a specific, logical structure. If you know where to look, you can ignore the white noise and find the signal.

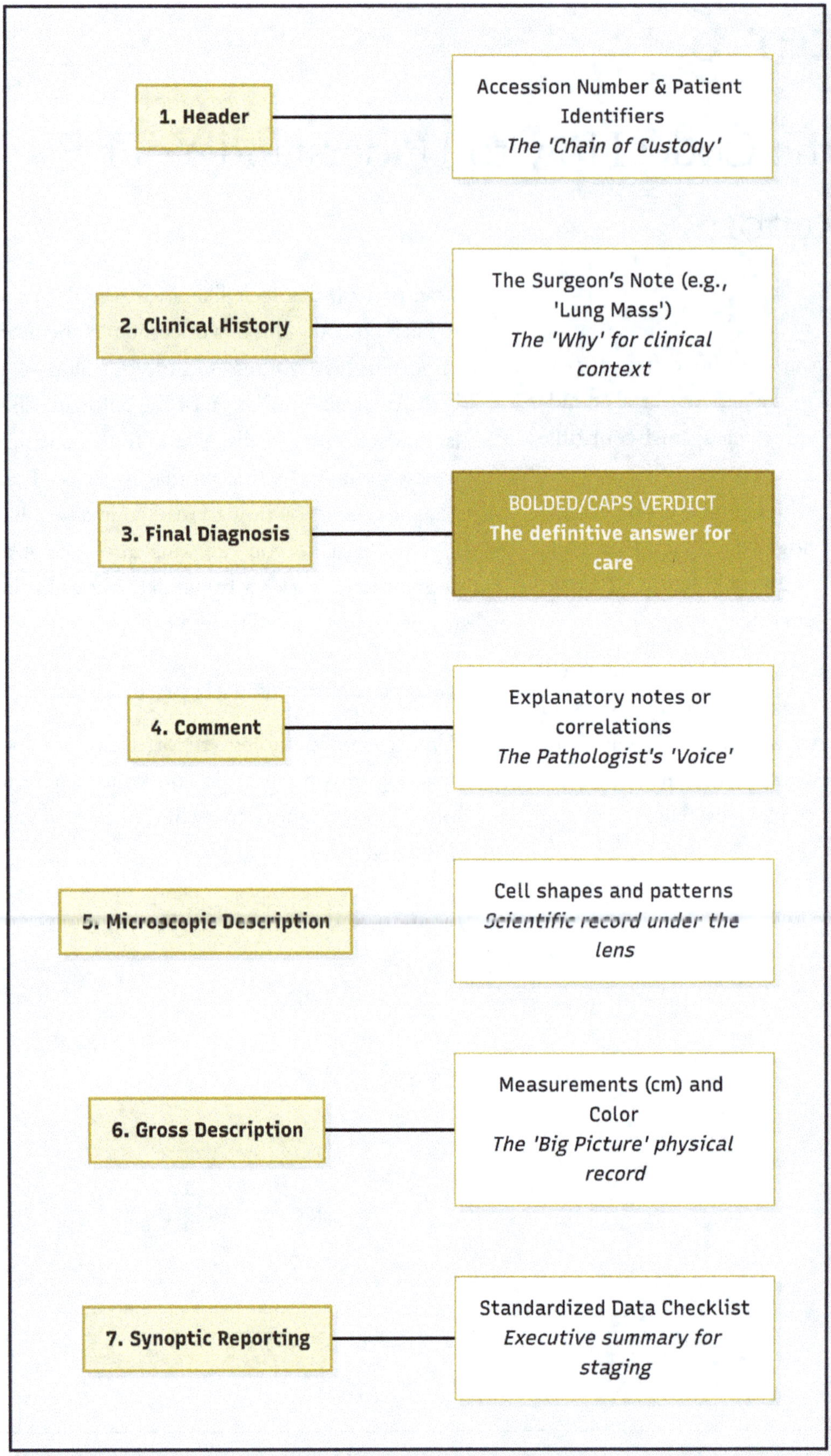
1. Header
Accession Number & Patient Identifiers
The 'Chain of Custody'
2. Clinical History
The Surgeon's Note (e.g., 'Lung Mass')
The 'Why' for clinical context
3. Final Diagnosis
BOLDED/CAPS VERDICT
The definitive answer for care
4. Comment
Explanatory notes or correlations
The Pathologist's 'Voice'
5. Microscopic Description
Cell shapes and patterns
Scientific record under the lens
6. Gross Description
Measurements (cm) and Color
The 'Big Picture' physical record
7. Synoptic Reporting
Standardized Data Checklist
Executive summary for staging

Fast & Reliable Results Concierge Service 24 Hour Support

DERMATOPATHOLOGY DIAGNOSTIC REPORT

Patient Details	Specimen Details	Ordering Provider	Guarantor
MRN: P DOB: Sex:	Accession: **LD24-** Procedure Date: Received Date: Reported Date:		

CLINICAL INFORMATION

A) Morphology: DDX: Neoplasm of Uncertain Behavior; Location: right anterior distal thigh;

DIAGNOSIS

SKIN, RIGHT ANTERIOR DISTAL THIGH, SHAVE REMOVAL:

- **MALIGNANT MELANOMA, AMELANOTIC, SUPERFICIAL SPREADING TYPE**
- **BRESLOW THICKNESS: 7.0MM**
- **CLARK'S LEVEL: AT LEAST IV**
- **MITOGENIC, TUMORIGENIC, ULCERATED**
- **MARGIN: POSITIVE DEEP AND PERIPHERAL**
- **PATHOLOGIC STAGE pT4b**

ICD 10: C43.71

Comment: Complete excision is recommended with adequate margins. IHC stains with Melan-A (+), SOX10 (+), HMB45 (+), and PRAME (90%) support the diagnosis.

DrHailu

Tesfu L Hailu, MD, FCAP, FASDP, FASCP, DABPath

MICROSCOPIC DESCRIPTION

The prominent histologic observations are nests of atypical melanocytes, and single melanocytes arranges in lentiginous fashion within the epidermis and at the dermal-epidermal junction. There is extension into the deep dermis in a nodular growth pattern where it involves the deep margins. There is an accompanying lymphohistiocytic infiltrate. Pigment is not present. The changes seen are those of amelanotic malignant melanoma. This would be a Clark's level IV/V lesion, measuring 7mm in thickness.

Hematoxylin-Eosin - right anterior distal thigh

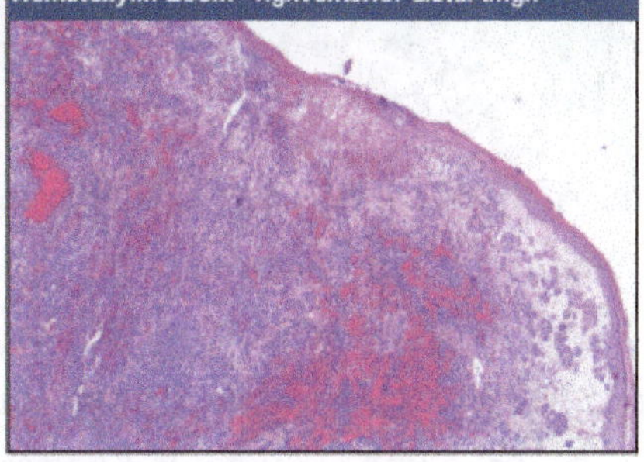

1. The Header (The Identification)

This is the specimen identification we discussed in Chapter 4 which contains items like your demographic information, the date of the procedure, and a unique Accession Number.

2. Clinical History (The Why)

This is a brief note from your surgeon to the pathologist. It might say, 55-year-old male with a 2cm lung mass, smoker. This is the context. It tells me what the clinical team was worried about before the microscopic characteristics of the biopsy was revealed.

3. Gross Description (The Macro)

Remember the Gross Room from Chapter 4? This is the record of what the tissue looked like to the naked eye. It will list the size, color, and/or weight.

Why it matters: If the surgeon removed a 5cm tumor, but the gross description says, Received a 2cm, it raises vital questions. Is it a partial/wedge biopsy or an erroneous data? Another question we ask is if the whole specimen was processed for microscopic examination, or just a piece of it.

4. Microscopic Description

Think of the Microscopic Description as the permanent, detailed record where I document the subtle nuances of your cells, the specific shape of the nuclei, the way the membranes interact, and the fine architectural patterns I observed under the lens. This is the foundational evidence of your case, written in the precise language of pathology. For simple benign cases, or biopsies of low grade malignancies, the report may have the diagnosis without microscopic description.

5. Synoptic Report

In a modern diagnostic report, the Synoptic Report acts as the executive summary that sits beneath the detailed Microscopic Description. It is not a replacement for the deep science, but a vital layer of protection to ensure nothing is lost in translation.

However, to ensure your surgical and oncology teams can act with lightning speed, we provide the Synoptic Report as a high-level, standardized checklist. This is a mission-critical data summary that lists the essential facts: the exact size of the tumor, the distance to the surgical margins, and whether the lymph nodes are involved, etc.

Synoptic Reporting is specialized. While it is the gold standard for most cancers, where specific data points like tumor grade and depth are used to determine your exact treatment plan, its only present on the reports of select specimen types.

For routine skin lesions or a simple infection, the traditional microscopic description provides all the information needed. We reserve the synoptic format for the complex cases where every millimeter and every metric carry the weight of a life-altering decision.

By layering these two formats, when necessary, we achieve a fail-safe communication style. The surgeon can find the vital statistics in seconds through the synoptic list, while the microscopic description remains as a comprehensive, scientific deep dive. This evolution in reporting ensures that the complexity of your biology is captured with absolute depth, while the path to your treatment remains clear, direct, and unambiguous.

6. The Final Diagnosis: The Verdict

The Final Diagnosis or simply Diagnosis is the most significant part of the pathology report. Usually located in a dedicated section or highlighted in bold, it carries the most diagnostic weight.

Everything else in the report, the gross description, measurements, microscopic findings, and special stains, serves as the supporting evidence. The Final Diagnosis is the formal conclusion drawn from that data. It is the medical verdict that guides clinical decisions and determines the next steps in a patient's care.

The Signature at the Bottom

Beneath the data and terminology is the signature of the pathologist, the physician who analyzed the cells and provided the final interpretation.

When you review your pathology report, engage with your medical team. Ask if the sample was adequate, whether the margins were clear, and if molecular or any necessary ancillary testing was performed. For complex or rare cases, requesting a subspecialty review is a standard commitment to diagnostic excellence.

You have now moved through the full journey of the biopsy: from the collection of tissue to the discovery of the truth.

The Dream and the Missing Specimen

A Personal Tale of Two Systems

Even for a trained pathologist, a modern laboratory can feel like a maze. During my fellowship in Surgical Pathology at the Hospital of the University of Pennsylvania, I experienced an event that I still describe as a miracle of the subconscious. I share this story not because it is dramatic, though it was, but because it reveals something essential about our work.

It had been a long day in the lab. I had received a breast core biopsy, reviewed the slides, finalized the diagnosis, and released out the report after it was signed by my attending pathologist. Once it disappeared into the digital ether, I did what every exhausted trainee does, I went home.

Around 7:30 PM that evening, just as I was beginning to unwind in my apartment, my pager shattered the quiet. When I returned the call, a surgical resident came on the line, sounding both urgent and confused.

Dr. Hailu, he said, I have the report for the breast biopsy, but we sent two specimens, the second specimen is a lymph node. It isn't in the report. What happened?

A cold wave of dread washed over me. In pathology, a missing specimen is the ultimate nightmare. It raises every terrifying possibility at once. Had it been lost in transit? Thrown away by mistake? Accessioned under a different number?

I explained that I was already home and promised I would investigate first thing in the morning. I took his contact information, hung up, and then discovered that my mind had no intention of resting.

That night, call it intuition, training, or the strange efficiency of the human mind under pressure, but I had a dream.

In the dream, I was in front of the laboratory information system, searching for the patient's lost specimen. But instead of navigating through Surgical Pathology, I found myself opening an entirely different module: Cytopathology.

Suddenly it became clear. The lymph node specimen wasn't a core of tissue at all. It was a Fine Needle Aspiration, a sample of cells rather than a solid piece of tissue. Because of that single technical distinction, it had been sent to a different division of the lab, processed by a different team, assigned a completely different tracking number, and results issued under a separate report by a cytopathologist.

In the dream, I opened the cytology report and read the words: Positive for adenocarcinoma. I also saw the name of the attending cytopathologist who signed the report at the bottom. I woke up stunned.

Somewhere between exhaustion and sleep, my subconscious had solved the puzzle my conscious mind had missed at the end of a long workday. Years of repetition had trained my brain to recognize the detail that mattered, that the lymph node was an FNA, even when fatigue had temporarily pushed it aside.

The moment I arrived at the hospital the next morning, I logged into the system. Exactly as I had seen in my dream, the axillary lymph node specimen was there within the cytopathology records. It had already been reviewed and signed out by the cytopathologist I see daily, exactly as I saw it. I immediately called the resident.

The specimen wasn't lost, I said, relief obvious in my voice. Because it was a Fine Needle Aspiration, it was processed as a cytology case in a different system. The report is finalized, and it confirms metastatic adenocarcinoma.

The case was closed. The panic resolved. But the lesson stayed with me.

The pathology laboratory is not a single hallway, it's an ecosystem. And sometimes, the answer resides at the intersection.

Anatomy and Cytology: Why Reports Split

Patients often ask a very reasonable question: Why isn't everything on one report?

In most large hospitals, the Department of Pathology is divided into several sub domains. Surgical Pathology handles solid pieces of tissue, biopsies, excisions, organ resections. These specimens undergo fixation, processing, embedding in wax, and microscopic slicing.

Cytopathology, on the other hand, deals with cells rather than tissue architecture. Fine needle aspirations, Pap smears, body fluids, and bronchial washings are processed differently, often spun in a centrifuge to make cell-blocks and also smeared directly onto slides.

Because these workflows require different equipment, different expertise, and sometimes even different computer systems, they generate separate reports. For patients, this can feel confusing or alarming.

But it is entirely normal for a needle biopsy and a surgical specimen from the same patient to result in two distinct diagnoses that arrive at different times.

The Subconscious Guardian

My experience at Penn taught me something that no textbook ever could: a pathologist is never truly off duty.

Our eyes are trained to recognize patterns, but our minds, and sometimes even our subconscious, are trained to protect the patient's story.

That instinct runs deeper than training alone. It is a constant, quiet vigilance. A reminder that behind every digital report and every glass slide is a human being whose well-being depends on careful attention.

Our work is not just about what we see under the microscope. It is about what must not be overlooked. We exist to make sure nothing important goes missing.

Chapter 7

Challenges of Biopsy

When Nothing Found Is Not the End of the Story

What False Negative Means

A biopsy is designed to answer a focused question. Most of the time, the answer is clear, and the result points confidently toward reassurance or treatment. A false negative result is different. It means that the biopsy did not show the problem that truly exists. In plain terms, the sample said no, but the person still has a condition that the diagnostic work did not capture.

This is not common, and it is never dismissed lightly. Modern biopsies are planned and performed to minimize the chance of missing a diagnosis. Even so, biology can be patchy, small targets can be elusive, and healing can temporarily erase clues. Understanding how and why a false negative can occur helps patients and clinicians respond wisely, without panic and without delay.

A false negative is not a failure of effort. It is a reminder that tissue is a snapshot, not a surveillance camera. The next step is to place that snapshot back into the whole story, symptoms, imaging, blood tests, and time, and decide whether to watch, to look again, or to change the approach.

Why It Happens

False negatives have a few recurring causes. The first and most common reason is inadequate sampling. Some diseases are focal, meaning they live in small islands inside otherwise normal tissue. If the needle or forceps land just beside the island, the sample can be entirely normal even though the target is real. This is why precise imaging guidance and careful mapping matter.

The second cause is biology. Certain conditions come and go. Inflammatory rashes or infections can wax and wane. A sample taken during a quiet moment may look normal, even though the pattern returns later. Tumors can also be heterogeneous, with aggressive areas next to quieter regions. If the sample comes from the quiet side, the most worrisome features may be missed.

A third contributor is processing. Pathology laboratories are designed to protect tissue and reveal detail, but very small or fragile samples can fragment. Crush artifact, cautery change, or scant cellularity can reduce what can be concluded with confidence. When that happens, pathologists say so plainly and recommend the safest next step.

Finally, there is interpretation and context. Pathology is not read in isolation. It is compared with imaging, procedure notes, and clinical history. If any piece does not fit, if the imaging looks dangerous and the tissue looks quiet, the team considers the tissue may not tell the full story and acts accordingly.

Where It Comes Up Most Often

A false negative result can appear in any organ, but the way it shows up varies. In the breast, tiny calcifications may represent early duct changes that require very specific targeting. If the cores do not include calcifications, radiologists and pathologists pause and often repeat the biopsy with a more focused approach. In the lung, small nodules can shift subtly with breathing; image guidance and post biopsy scans help confirm that the true target was sampled. In the prostate, cancer often grows in small foci or in the front part of the gland; that is why modern approaches include MRI targeted sampling and trans-perineal routes to reach difficult areas.

In the gastrointestinal tract, flat lesions can hide in folds, and inflammatory diseases can skip from patch to patch. Multiple small biopsies from mapped locations create a better picture than a single sample. In the skin and mouth, the most informative piece is often taken from the edge of a changing area, where normal meets abnormal and the diagnosis declares itself. In bone marrow, the liquid aspirate and the solid core answer different questions; sometimes one is diagnostic when the other is not, and both are needed to see the whole process.

Across these settings, the pattern is the same. When the team deliberately matches the sampling method to the biology of the disease, false negative results become uncommon, though never impossible.

How Teams Minimize the Risk

Pre procedure planning is the first active risk reduction step. Radiologists, surgeons, and pathologists agree on the question being asked and the target being sampled. If muscle must be present in a bladder specimen to judge depth, the procedure aims to include it. If a liver disease needs a minimum length of core to compare portal tracts, the plan reflects that requirement. When an endometrial biopsy must reach enough lining to be trustworthy, adequacy is front of mind from the start.

During the procedure, precision and adequacy are actively monitored. Imaging guidance confirms trajectory and location. When feasible, on site assessment checks that a sample contains the expected cells before the procedure ends. The number of cores is chosen to balance safety with confidence; sometimes a few more samples mean a great deal fewer questions later.

After the procedure, radiology pathology correlation closes the loop. The pathologist reviews the slides with the radiologist's description in hand. If the report says negative but the imaging screamed suspicious, that discordance is not ignored. It triggers a phone call, a conference, or a repeat sample.

Words in the Report That Signal Caution

Pathology reports use consistent language to communicate confidence. Negative for malignancy is a clear statement, but it lives inside context. If the report also notes that the sample was scant, fragmented, or limited by artifact, your clinician will factor that into next steps. Phrases like nondiagnostic or insufficient for evaluation are flags that may indicate that the tissue was not enough to answer the question.

What the Report Says	What it Means in Plain English	Why it Happens
Scant cellularity	Not enough cells to be sure.	The needle or swab didn't pick up enough material to provide a representative sample.
Crush artifact	The cells were squeezed; we can't see detail.	Cells are fragile; if they are compressed during collection or processing, their structures distort.
Nondiagnostic	This sample didn't answer the question.	A catch-all term meaning the lab cannot give a definitive yes or no based on what was sent.

Sometimes the report uses words such as atypical or suspicious. These terms mean that some features pointed toward a significant diagnosis, but not enough were present to be definitive. In these situations, the safest path is often to repeat the biopsy, sample a different area, or use a different technique. These terms are protective. They prevent over calling on thin evidence and under calling when danger is possible.

When Watchful Waiting Is Wise, and When It Isn't

Time can be a powerful diagnostic tool. Many negative biopsies are followed by calm observation because the full story, imaging, exam, and symptoms, supports that choice. A reactive lymph node after a viral illness, a skin rash that is already improving, or a breast finding classified as low suspicion may all be managed with short interval follow up. If the picture stays quiet, the negative biopsy gets corroborated by reality.

Other times, waiting is not the right answer. If a lesion grows, if symptoms escalate, or if the imaging and the biopsy do not agree, doing nothing can carry risk. In those moments, repeating the biopsy, choosing a larger sample, or proceeding to removal is the safer path. The distinction is not made by fear; it is made by fit. When evidence aligns, watching is wise. When evidence conflicts, looking again is prudent.

Changing the Approach Can Change the Answer

If a first biopsy misses the mark, the second does not have to repeat the same plan. Imaging can be upgraded from ultrasound to MRI.

The route can shift from trans-rectal to trans-perineal to reach a hard to sample region. A fine needle aspiration can give way to a core, or a core to an excision. In the GI tract, additional mapped biopsies or removal of a polyp at its base may be more informative than another superficial pinch.

These changes are deliberate adjustments designed to answer the original question with greater certainty and less room for doubt.

What Pathologists Do Behind the Scenes

Pathologists review the clinical history, procedure notes, and imaging impressions. They decide whether deeper sections are needed from the tissue block to search for a small focus that was not visible at first sections/cuts. They add special stains or molecular tests when those tools can turn uncertainty into clarity. If a result could change management, a second pathologist often reviews the slides. This internal consultation is built into routine practice because the stakes justify the time.

When the language in a report signals a limitation, it is the result of this careful process. The words are chosen to convey exactly how trustworthy the conclusion is so that clinicians can match the next step to the level of confidence.

Safety Nets You Can See and Feel

From the patient's perspective, safety looks like a plan. After a negative biopsy, clinicians set a timeline for follow up that fits the level of concern. Imaging is repeated according to the standard interval. Symptoms are revisited and new information is compared with the original findings. If the story changes, the plan changes too.

Good plans also survive hand offs. Your primary clinician, radiologist, surgeon, and pathologist share information so that no single piece of the puzzle gets lost. You may also receive a copy of your report and your follow up schedule in writing, which lets you know what will happen and when, and gives you a clear point of contact if something changes sooner than expected.

Short Vignettes That Show the Process Working

A small cluster of calcifications appeared on a screening mammogram. The first biopsy cores did not contain calcifications on the specimen X ray, and the pathology report was benign but limited. The radiologist requested a repeat biopsy with stereotactic targeting. The second set included calcifications, and the pathology revealed an early, highly treatable lesion. The limited first result became a steppingstone for the subsequent diagnosis.

A coin sized lung nodule was biopsied with a fine needle, and the result showed only inflammation. Because the nodule looked suspicious on CT and the patient's symptoms persisted, the team repeated the procedure with a thicker core needle under CT guidance. This time, the sample captured the true process, and treatment began promptly.

A prostate biopsy showed low grade cancer in only one small core. The PSA, however, continued to rise steadily, and MRI suggested a lesion in the front of the gland that standard sampling can miss. A transperineal, MRI targeted biopsy found a higher grade focus. The plan shifted from watchful waiting to treatment guided by the more accurate picture.

Questions Worth Asking

After a negative or limited biopsy, it is reasonable to ask how well the sample matched the target. You can ask whether the tissue contained the features that imaging suggested should be present. You can ask whether enough tissue was obtained to be confident and what limitations, if any, the pathologist noted. You can ask what signs or timing would prompt a repeat biopsy, a different technique, or a definitive removal.

These are not adversarial questions. They are the same questions your care team asks one another behind the scenes. When you ask them, you join the conversation and help ensure that the plan fits your condition.

What This Means for You

A biopsy that says no cancer is usually exactly what it seems: a relief backed by evidence. When results do not fit the rest of the story, the answer is not to worry without action or to act without thought. The answer is to reconnect the tissue with the imaging, the symptoms, and time, and then choose the next step intentionally.

False negative results are the exception, not the rule. When they occur, they are met with safeguards, planning, precision, correlation, and follow up. The process is designed to protect the patient from both over treatment and under treatment.

With that understanding, the next step is no longer guesswork. If the right answer was not visible today, the plan makes sure it will be visible tomorrow, before it has the chance to cause harm.

If you remember one simple script for every pathology report, it is this: what did you find, how certain are you, what are my options, and why is this option right for me? Those four questions turn an intimidating document into a manageable conversation, and they work for every biopsy in every chapter that follows. With those answers, decisions become informed, and care becomes collaborative.

Across every organ in the chapters ahead, biopsies serve the same purpose. Whether the tissue comes from the lung, liver, kidney, bladder, or anywhere else, the goal is the same: to replace uncertainty with a plan.

Part II

The Language of the Lens, Navigating the Most Common Biopsies

A Shared Journey: Understanding the Scale of Diagnostic Truth

If you're waiting for biopsy results, you're not alone. You're part of a vast global community of people seeking clarity about their health. The data in the table below highlights the enormous scale of modern pathology, millions of patients undergoing similar diagnostic harvests every year. Statistics from trusted organizations such as the National Institute of Diabetes and Digestive and Kidney Diseases (NIDDK) and the Skin Cancer Foundation remind us that biopsies remain one of the most essential tools in medicine, used to safeguard countless lives.

Although the true scale is unknown, since not all data are centralized or consistently reported, the volume of biopsies performed each year offers a sense of the enormous collective effort to turn uncertainty into answers. From an estimated 20 million gastrointestinal biopsies each year to roughly 10 million skin samples examined annually, these numbers represent millions of patients seeking answers and millions of clinicians working to provide it.

The sheer volume can seem overwhelming, but most of these procedures end with reassuring news. For example, of the approximately 1.5 million breast biopsies performed each year to evaluate a concerning finding, about 80% return benign results, a statistic that underscores how often a biopsy rules out, rather than confirms, a feared diagnosis.

Whether it's a gentle thyroid whisper or a precisely guided lung biopsy, each procedure is backed by the expertise of organizations like the American Cancer Society (ACS) and the American Thyroid Association (ATA). Behind every data point lies a person who took a courageous step toward getting an answer to a problem. By participating in this process, you're giving your medical team the key needed to open a locked door, bringing you one step closer to your own answer.

Table: Annual Biopsies Performed in the USA by Category

Category	Est. Annual	Primary Driver	Key Source
GI	20,000,000	Colonoscopies/EGDs (Polyps, H. pylori)	*NIDDK / iData*
Skin	10,000,000	Melanoma, Basal Cell, Benign Lesions	*Medicare / SCF*
Breast	1,500,000	Abnormal Mammography (80% Benign)	*NCHR / CMS*
Endometrial	1,000,000	Post-menopausal/Abnormal Bleeding	*ACOG / ACS*
Prostate	1,000,000	Elevated PSA / MRI-Fusion Targeting	*UCLA / USPSTF*
Cervical	750,000	Abnormal Pap/HPV Follow-up	*ASCCP*
Thyroid	700,000	FNA of Ultrasound-detected Nodules	*ATA / BD*
Oral Cavity	350,000	Persistent Sores or White Patches	*ADA / SEER*
Lung	250,000	Low-Dose CT Smoker Screening	*ACR Registry*
Lymph Nodes	250,000	Cancer Staging / Lymphoma Suspicion	*SEER*
Bladder	180,000	Hematuria Investigation/Monitoring	*AUA*
Kidney	100,000	Renal Masses / Transplant Health	*AUA*
Liver	70,000	NASH/MASH or Tumor Diagnostics	*AASLD*
Bone Marrow	65,000	Leukemia, Myeloma, Anemia	*LLS / SEER*
Pancreas	55,000	High-Complexity EUS Biopsies	*ASGE*
Vulvar	45,000	Chronic Skin Conditions / VIN	*ACOG*
Penis	25,000	Lichen Sclerosus/BXO, PeIN, carcinoma	*ACS/ISPOR*
TOTAL	**~36.2M+**	**Aggregated Tissue Samples**	*Grand View / SkyQuest*

Organ and Tissue Specific Biopsies

The next several chapters are dedicated to individual biopsy types. You're welcome to read them all or simply focus on the ones most relevant to you. Think of this section as a reference you can return to whenever you need clarity or reassurance.

Although the laboratory process, preserving, processing, slicing, and staining tissue, is standardized across all biopsy types, the questions each biopsy answers depend entirely on where the sample comes from. What matters in a skin biopsy is different from what matters in the colon, the breast, or the prostate.

Consider this your field guide to the biopsies most commonly performed in the world, written to demystify every step from procedure to pathology report.

Note: These chapters are educational and general. They are not designed to be exhaustive but instead as clear, concise, simple, and helpful as possible. Your own clinicians know your medical history and will tailor medical advice to your specific situation. This book is not a substitute for professional medical guidance.

Chapter 8

Gastrointestinal (GI) Biopsies

Small Samples That Explain Symptoms and Prevent Cancer

What It Is and Why It's Done

Gastrointestinal biopsies are very small samples taken from the lining of the digestive tract. During procedures such as colonoscopy or upper endoscopy, doctors may take tiny pinch samples from the inner lining of the esophagus, stomach, small intestine, colon, or rectum. These samples are collected using delicate instruments passed through the scope, and most people do not feel them at all.

These small samples help explain symptoms that cannot be fully understood from imaging or blood/stool tests alone. Bleeding, abdominal pain, anemia, chronic diarrhea, or changes in bowel habits often leave subtle clues at the tissue level. Under the microscope, biopsies can reveal inflammation, infection, irritation, or early cellular changes that are invisible during the procedure itself.

GI biopsies are also central to cancer prevention. Their main contribution is identifying polyps — small growths along the digestive tract. While many polyps are harmless, some can slowly progress into cancer over time. Finding and removing these changes early dramatically reduces the risk of cancer occurring later.

But GI biopsies are not limited to colon polyps. Gastric biopsies from the stomach are frequently taken to diagnose H. pylori infection, evaluate ulcers, and rule out malignancy when symptoms or endoscopic findings raise concern. These small samples help determine the cause of chronic stomach pain, inflammation, or bleeding, often leading to targeted treatment that prevents future complications.

Similarly, esophageal biopsies are essential for identifying conditions such as Barrett's esophagus, a precancerous change associated with long-standing acid reflux, and eosinophilic esophagitis, an allergy-related inflammatory disorder. These diagnoses cannot be made by appearance alone, they require microscopic confirmation. Catching them early guides treatment and, in the case of Barrett's, can reduce the risk of esophageal cancer.

Although GI biopsies are tiny, their impact is significant. They help explain symptoms, guide treatment, and often prevent serious disease before it has the chance to develop. For many patients, this process turns an uncertain situation into a clear and manageable plan.

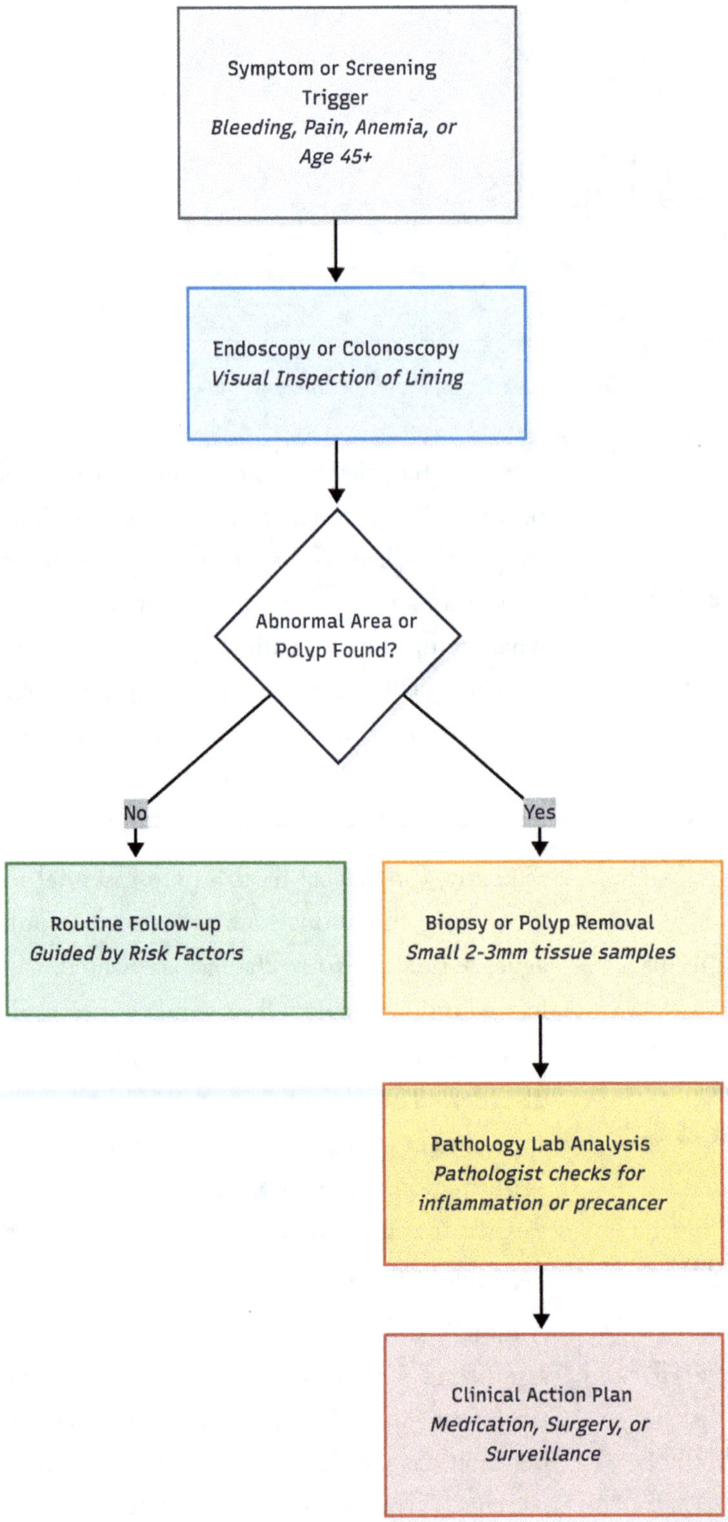

How the Biopsy Is Performed

During a colonoscopy or upper endoscopy, most patients are sedated and comfortable. A thin, flexible camera is gently guided through the digestive tract, allowing the gastroenterologist to carefully inspect the lining of the esophagus, stomach, or colon. If an area looks abnormal, or even slightly unusual, very small tissue samples are taken. These samples are usually only a few millimeters in size.

Polyps are commonly removed during the same procedure. Removing them at this stage is both diagnostic and preventive, as it allows the tissue to be examined while also eliminating a potential future problem. These procedures are typically outpatient, meaning patients go home the same day once the sedation has worn off.

Although most people feel alert afterward, sedation can continue to affect judgment and reflexes longer than expected. For safety, patients are advised not to drive, operate machinery, or make important decisions for the rest of the day. Most facilities require a responsible adult to accompany patients home after the procedure.

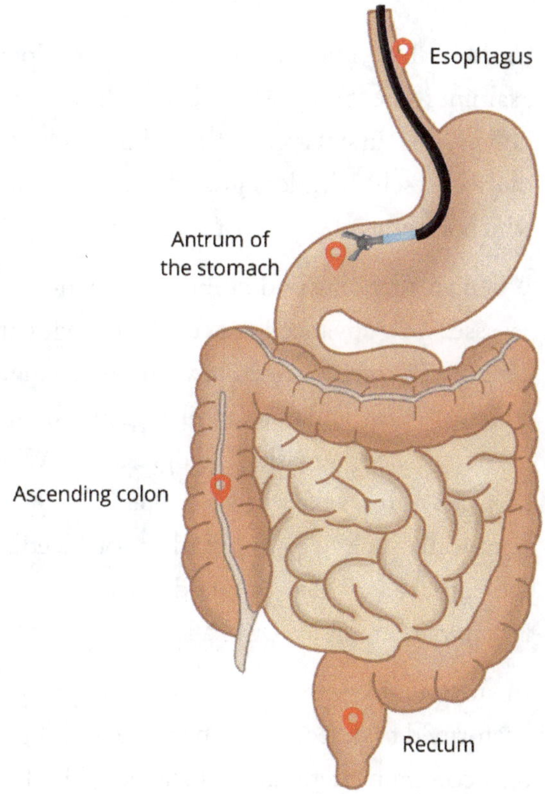

Figure 5. Endoscopic biopsy

In the Pathology Laboratory

In the pathology laboratory, biopsy samples arrive in several small containers, each carefully labeled according to where the tissue was taken. Labels might specify areas such as the stomach, different parts of the colon, or a particular polyp.

Each location is processed separately. This allows the final pathology report to serve as a precise map of the digestive tract. When your doctor reviews the report with you, each diagnosis corresponds to a specific location, helping guide accurate treatment decisions and follow up planning.

What the Pathologist Looks For

Under the microscope, the pathologist examines the tissue at a cellular level. For polyps, the first task is determining whether they represent harmless growths or adenomas, which are true precancerous lesions.

When an adenoma is identified, the pathologist assesses how advanced the cellular changes are. These can range from low grade changes, which are early and mild, to high grade changes that carry a higher risk of progression. When biopsies are taken to evaluate ongoing symptoms such as pain, diarrhea, or bleeding, the focus shifts toward patterns of inflammation, injury, or healing.

In stomach biopsies, additional testing may be performed to detect Helicobacter pylori (figure 6), a common bacterium associated with ulcers and chronic inflammation. When detected, these organisms will look brown or red against a light blue background.

How Results Are Reported

Your report will name what was found in specific terms and indicate how concerning it is. The diagnostic phrases you will see are designed to distinguish between changes that need only monitoring and those that need closer follow-up or treatment. These terms help doctors distinguish between changes that require routine monitoring and those that need closer follow up or treatment.

When the diagnosis is cancer, most commonly a type called adenocarcinoma in the gastrointestinal tract, the report clearly names it and outlines the key features needed to guide care. These details help determine the stage of the disease, the appropriate treatment options, and the next steps in management.

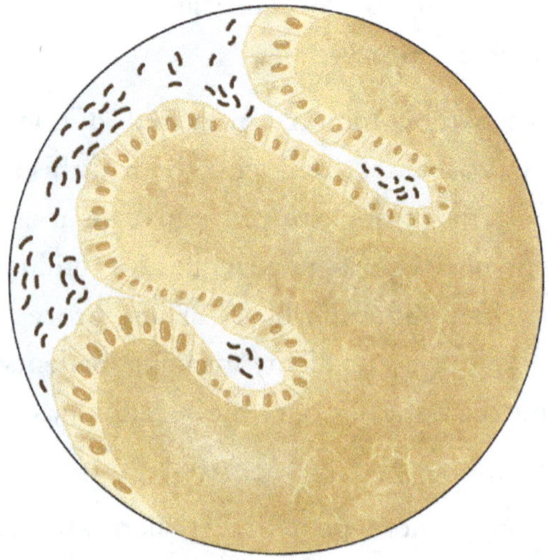

Figure 6. Helicobacter pylori bacteria seen on the lining of the stomach.

What Happens Next

When biopsies show benign tissue or low risk findings, no further treatment may be necessary beyond routine follow up. If inflammation or infection is identified, treatment may include medications, dietary changes, or management of an underlying condition.

When polyps are removed, the type and features of the polyp determine when the next colonoscopy should be performed. This personalized planning ensures that follow up is neither too frequent nor too delayed and that prevention remains effective over time.

Common Fears and Reassurances

The word polyp lands hard on a patient. I have read enough of my own reports back to know that almost no one hears "tubular adenoma, completely excised" the way the pathologist intended it. They hear cancer. What they should hear is the opposite. Most of the polyps that come across my desk are the medical equivalent of a smoke detector going off because a piece of toast got too close. The detector did its job. Someone unplugged the toaster. The house is fine.

What makes colon screening unusual, almost gentle by the standards of cancer medicine, is the runway. A typical adenoma takes a decade or more to drift toward malignancy. That is a long time to catch it, and we usually do. By the time you are reading the report, the small growth has often already been snared off the wall of your colon, dropped into formalin, and on its way to my microscope. The disease the polyp might have become, ten or fifteen years from now, has been quietly prevented.

The Five Step Path From Polyp to Colon Cancer

The inner lining of the colon is made of cells that grow, shed, and regenerate on a rapid cycle. This fast turnover keeps the tissue healthy and functioning properly. However, the same rapid renewal also makes these cells more vulnerable to mutations, simply because they divide so often. In the earliest stages, everything still appears completely normal under the microscope.

Over time, a disruption in growth control can lead to the formation of a small adenomatous polyp. Under the microscope, cells may appear slightly crowded or disorganized but remain confined to the surface lining.

Some adenomatous polyps continue to grow and develop more concerning features. These advanced adenomatous polyps may be larger or show more abnormal cell architecture. We call these adenomatous polyp with high-grade dysplasia. Although they are still not cancer, their risk of progression is higher if left untreated.

In the next stage, cancer cells are forming but remain limited to the innermost layers of the polyp. We call these carcinoma in-situ. These early cancers are highly treatable.

If the process continues unchecked, cancer cells can invade deeper layers and spread beyond the colon. Screening aims to interrupt this progression long before this stage is reached.

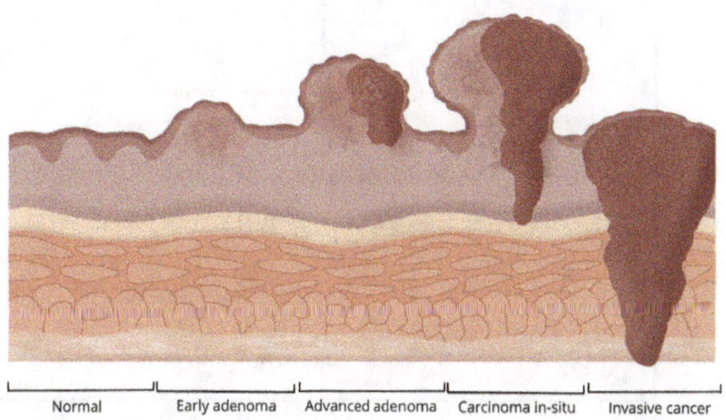

Figure 7. Progression of normal colon lining to adenomatous polyp, adenomatous polyp with high grade dysplasia, and finally to colon cancer (in-situ and invasive).

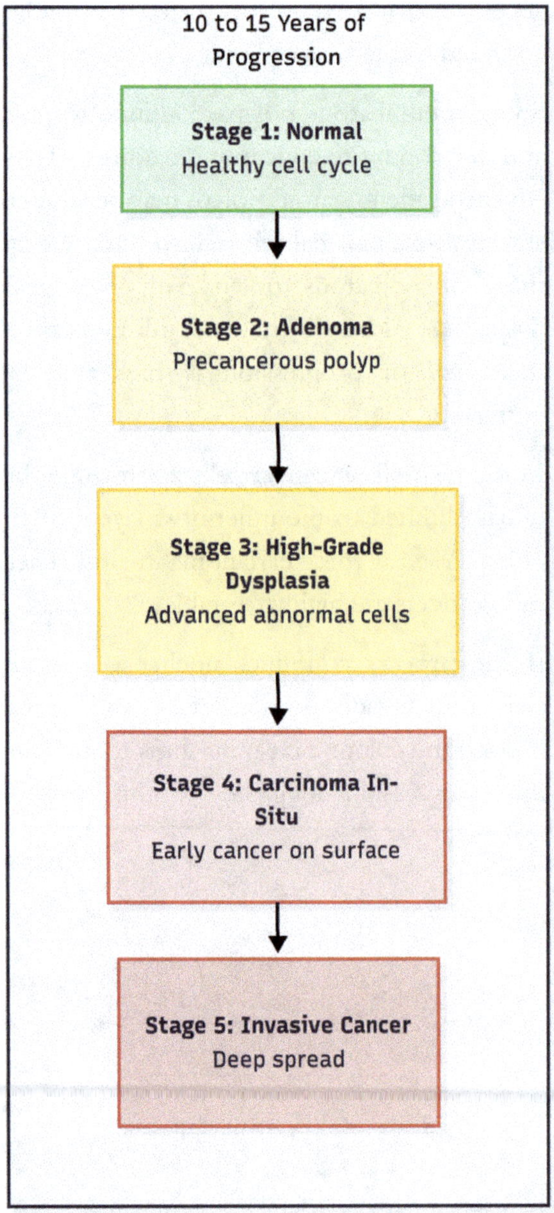

How Pathology Findings Guide Future Screenings

Pathology results play a central role in determining when the next colonoscopy should occur. National guidelines are used to personalize follow up intervals based on risk.

Low risk findings often allow long intervals between exams, sometimes many years. Higher risk features lead to earlier follow up to ensure that new changes are caught at a treatable stage. This balance avoids unnecessary procedures while maintaining strong cancer prevention.

When inflammation or infection is identified, pathology results guide medication choices, dietary recommendations, and other aspects of care. In this way, GI biopsy findings become a practical roadmap rather than just a diagnosis.

Example

During a routine screening colonoscopy, a small polyp is detected and removed. Pathology shows it is a benign adenomatous polyp with early, low-grade changes. Because it was completely removed, the risk of transformation into cancer is eliminated. The follow up schedule is adjusted appropriately, and a potential future problem is quietly prevented years before it could cause harm.

> 💡 **Author Tip: The 'Prep' and the 'Yield'**
>
> **A Clean View for a Clear Sample:** The quality of your bowel prep directly affects biopsy accuracy.
>
> If the doctor can't clearly see the lining, small polyps or subtle abnormalities can be missed.
>
> A thorough prep ensures every millimeter is inspected and sampled correctly.

What This Means for You

GI biopsies are small, but their value is substantial. They explain symptoms, guide treatment, and prevent cancer through early detection and removal of precancerous changes. When combined with thoughtful follow up, they replace uncertainty with a planned management.

Rather than creating alarm, the process produces a schedule. The biopsy result tells your gastroenterologist when to see you next — three years, five, ten — and that schedule, more than anything else, is what keeps colon cancer from forming in the first place.

Questions to Ask Your Doctor During a Follow-up Appointment

On the Results and Findings

1. What was the specific type of polyp or tissue found? (e.g., Was it a tubular adenoma, hyperplastic polyp, or sessile serrated lesion?)
2. Were there any signs of high-grade dysplasia?
3. Did the biopsy confirm a specific cause for my symptoms? (Does the report show infection, H. pylori, or inflammation like Celiac disease or IBD?)

On Future Prevention

1. Based on these results, when is my next colonoscopy or endoscopy due? (Ask for a specific year based on the pathology findings.)
2. Was the entire polyp or lesion removed during the procedure?
3. Does this diagnosis change my risk profile for the future?
4. Do my family members need to be screened earlier because of this finding?

On Treatment and Recovery

1. Do I need to start any new medications or change my diet based on these results?
2. Are there any activities I should still avoid as the biopsy sites finish healing?

Recommended GI Exam Protocol

Gastroenterologists follow a protocol based on age, risk factors, and previous pathology findings.

Upper GI (Endoscopy) Monitoring

- Upper GI endoscopies are usually performed to investigate specific symptoms (like GERD or difficulty swallowing).
- If a biopsy shows Barrett's Esophagus (a change in the lining of the esophagus), the protocol shifts to regular surveillance every 3 to 5 years to prevent esophageal cancer.

Colonoscopy Screening Timeline

- Average Risk: For those with no family history, the universal recommendation for a first screening colonoscopy is age 45.
- Earlier Screening: If you have a first-degree relative (parent or sibling) with colon cancer or polyps, screening typically begins at age 40, or 10 years younger than the age at which the relative was diagnosed.

The 10-Year Gold Standard

If a colonoscopy is clean (no polyps found and no family history), the universal interval for the next exam is 10 years. However, this could change based on biopsy findings:

- 1 - 2 Small Adenomas: Usually results in a repeat exam in 5 to 10 years.
- 3 or More Adenomas (or High-Grade Dysplasia): Usually requires a repeat exam in 3 years.
- Incomplete Removal: May require a follow-up in 6 months to 1 year.

The Symptom-Driven Protocol

Regardless of when your last clear exam was, the protocol dictates an immediate evaluation if you experience Alarm Symptoms:

- Rectal bleeding or blood in the stool.
- Unexplained weight loss or anemia.
- A persistent change in bowel habits lasting more than a few weeks.

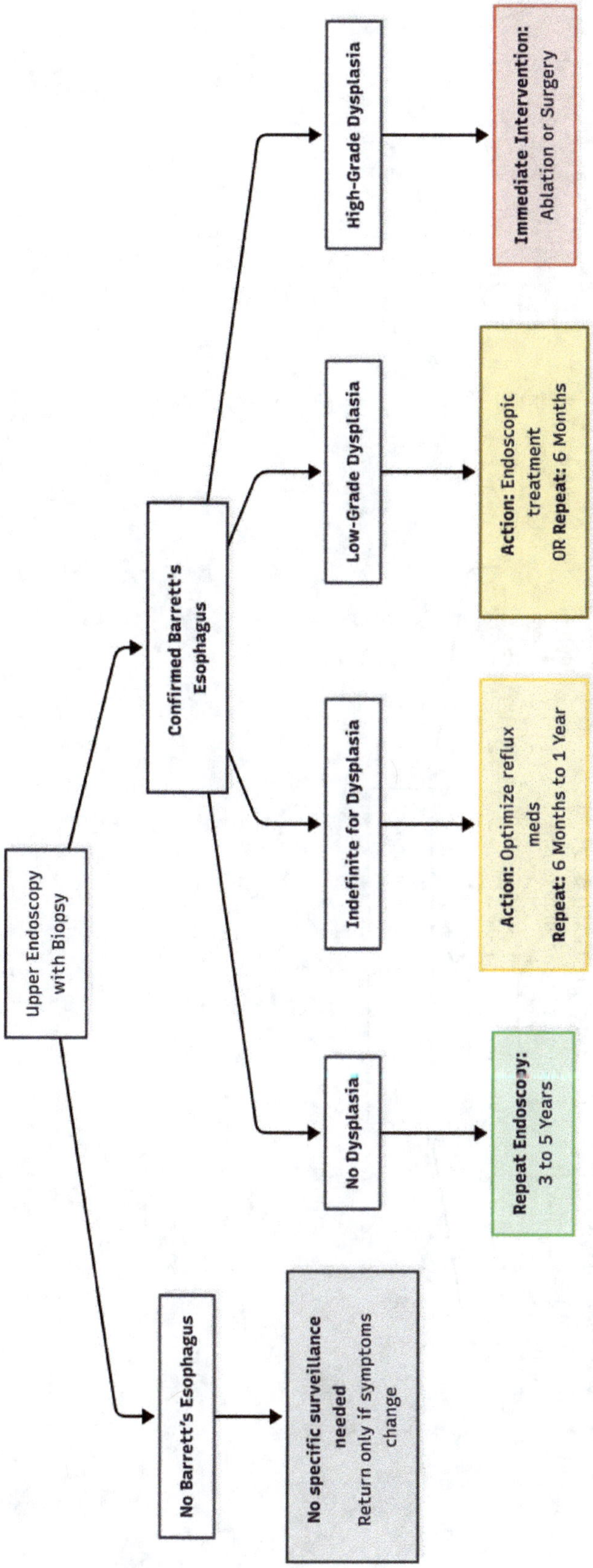

Upper GI Endoscopy Flowchart

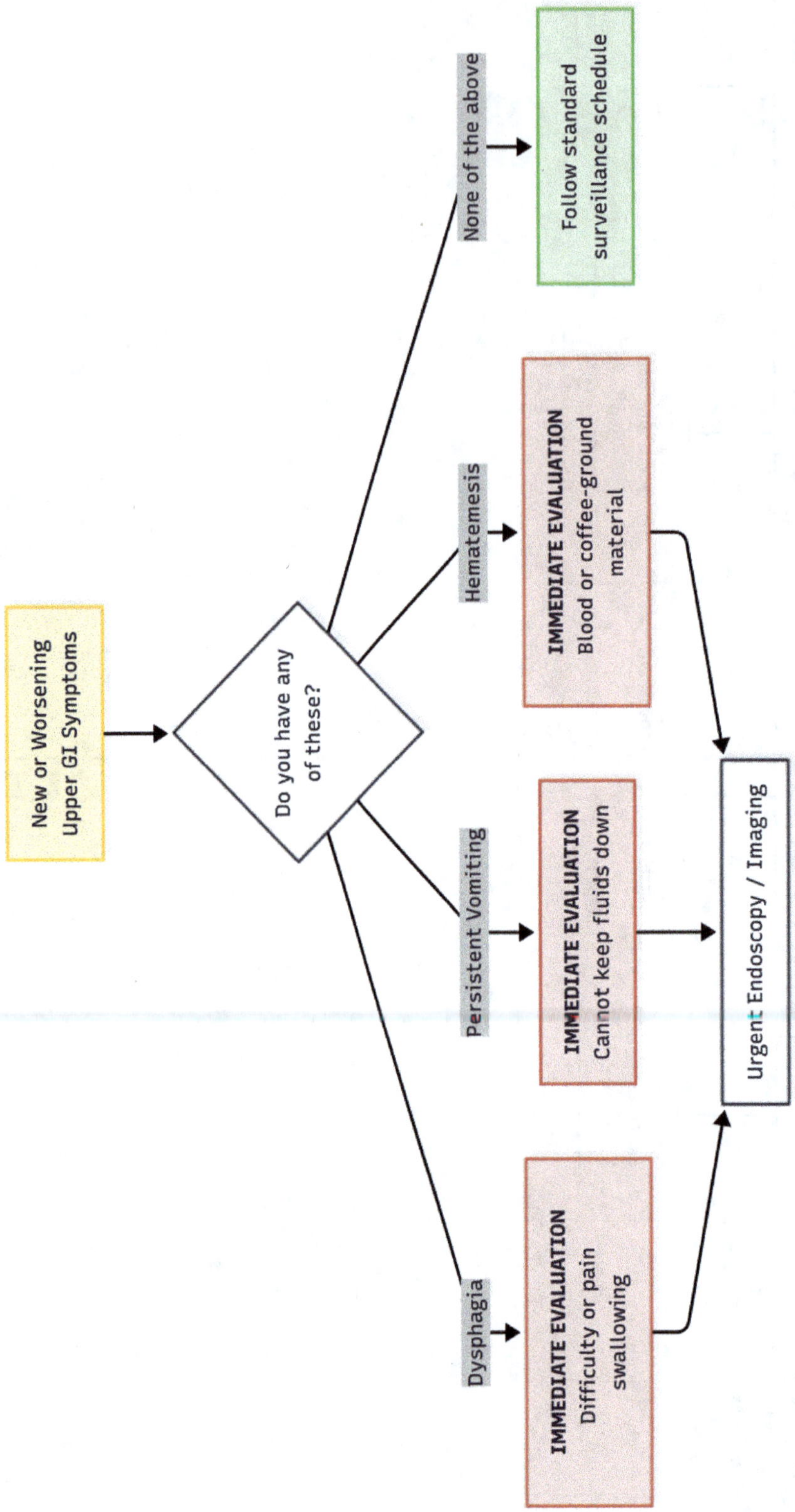

The Alarm Protocol for Upper GI

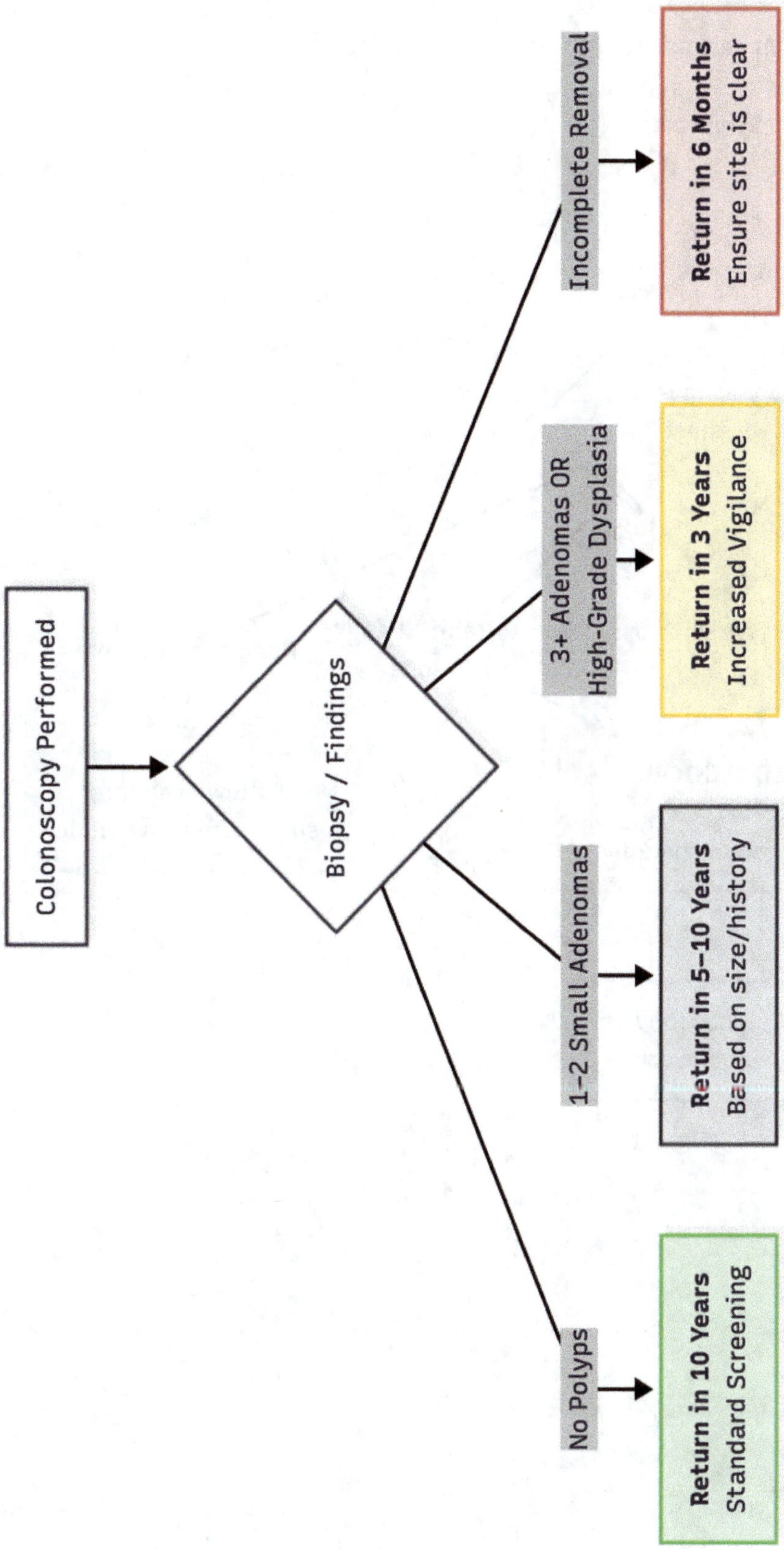

Colonoscopy Biopsy Result Flowchart

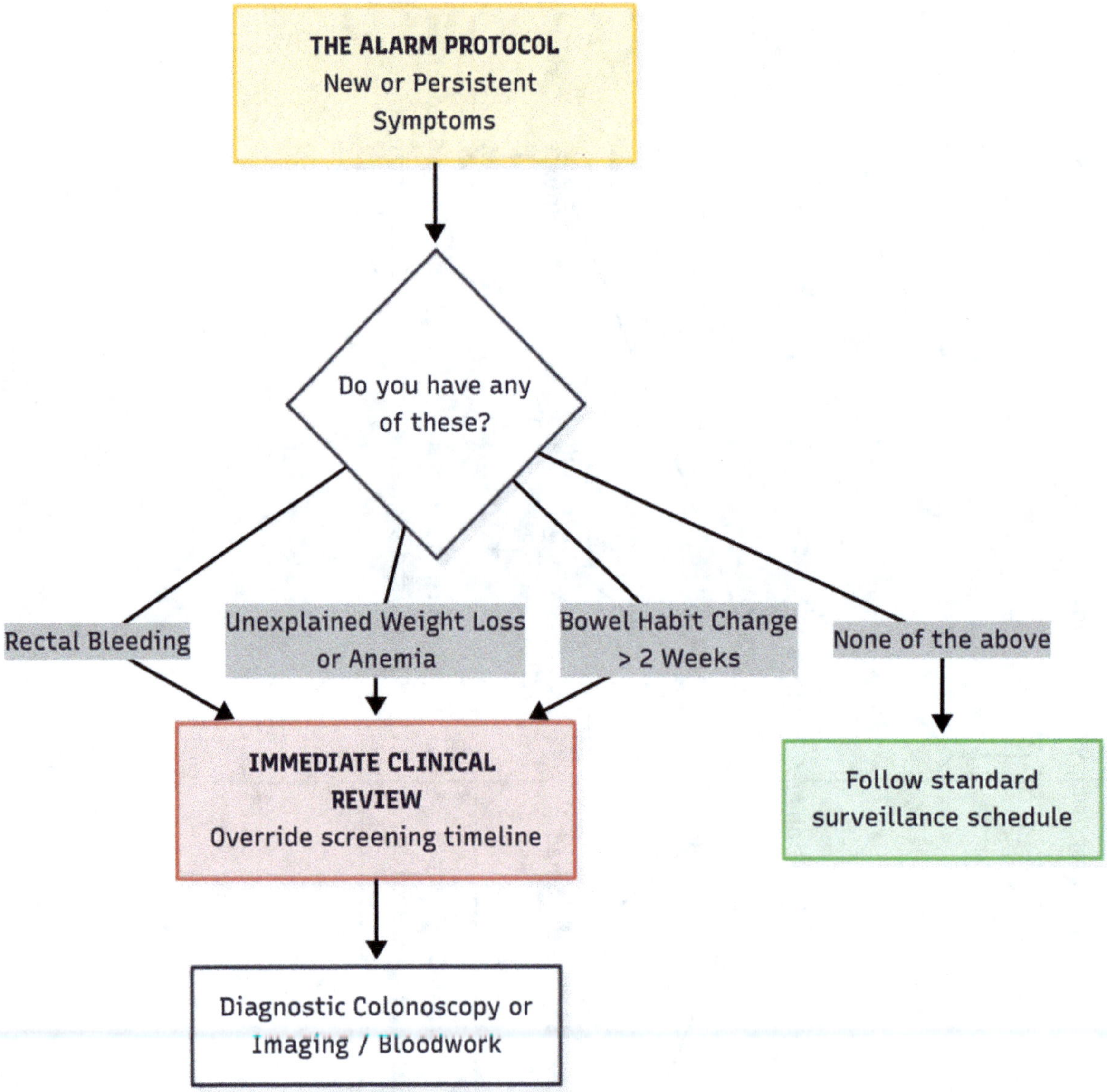

Colonoscopy Alarm Protocol Flowchart

Quick Summary

- A GI biopsy is a tiny pinch sample from the digestive tract lining — usually painless and taken during a colonoscopy or endoscopy you are already sedated for.
- The biopsy answers two kinds of questions: what is causing unexplained symptoms (bleeding, pain, reflux), and is a polyp benign, precancerous, or an early cancer.
- Colon cancer develops slowly over 10–15 years through a predictable polyp-to-cancer sequence. Finding and removing polyps interrupts that pathway before cancer can form.
- Your follow-up interval (3, 5, or 10 years) is set by what the biopsy shows. The pathology result personalizes your next colonoscopy date, not your age.
- Arrange a ride home and skip major decisions for 24 hours after sedation, even if you feel alert.

Chapter 9

Skin Biopsies

Understanding Spots, Rashes, and Moles

What It Is and Why It's Done

A skin biopsy removes a very small piece of skin to explain a spot, rash, or mole that has changed, persisted, or looks unusual. The goal is to understand what the visually observed finding on the skin truly shows under the microscope. Some changes are harmless. Others reflect inflammation, infection, or irritation. A small number represent early changes that could be precancerous or cancer.

Because the skin, the largest organ, and is readily visible, people often notice changes early. That visibility is an advantage. A biopsy allows your care team to move from visual concern to biological certainty and decide whether reassurance, treatment, or simple monitoring is the right next step.

How the Biopsy Is Performed

The procedure begins by numbing the area to make you as comfortable as possible during the procedure. Once the skin is numb, your clinician removes a small sample. Depending on the situation, this may be a tiny core of skin, a thin surface layer, or sometimes the entire spot. The choice depends on what is being evaluated and where it is located.

Most skin biopsies take only a few minutes. Some require a stitch, but many do not. Afterward, the area is covered and simple care instructions are given. Normal activities can usually be resumed quickly.

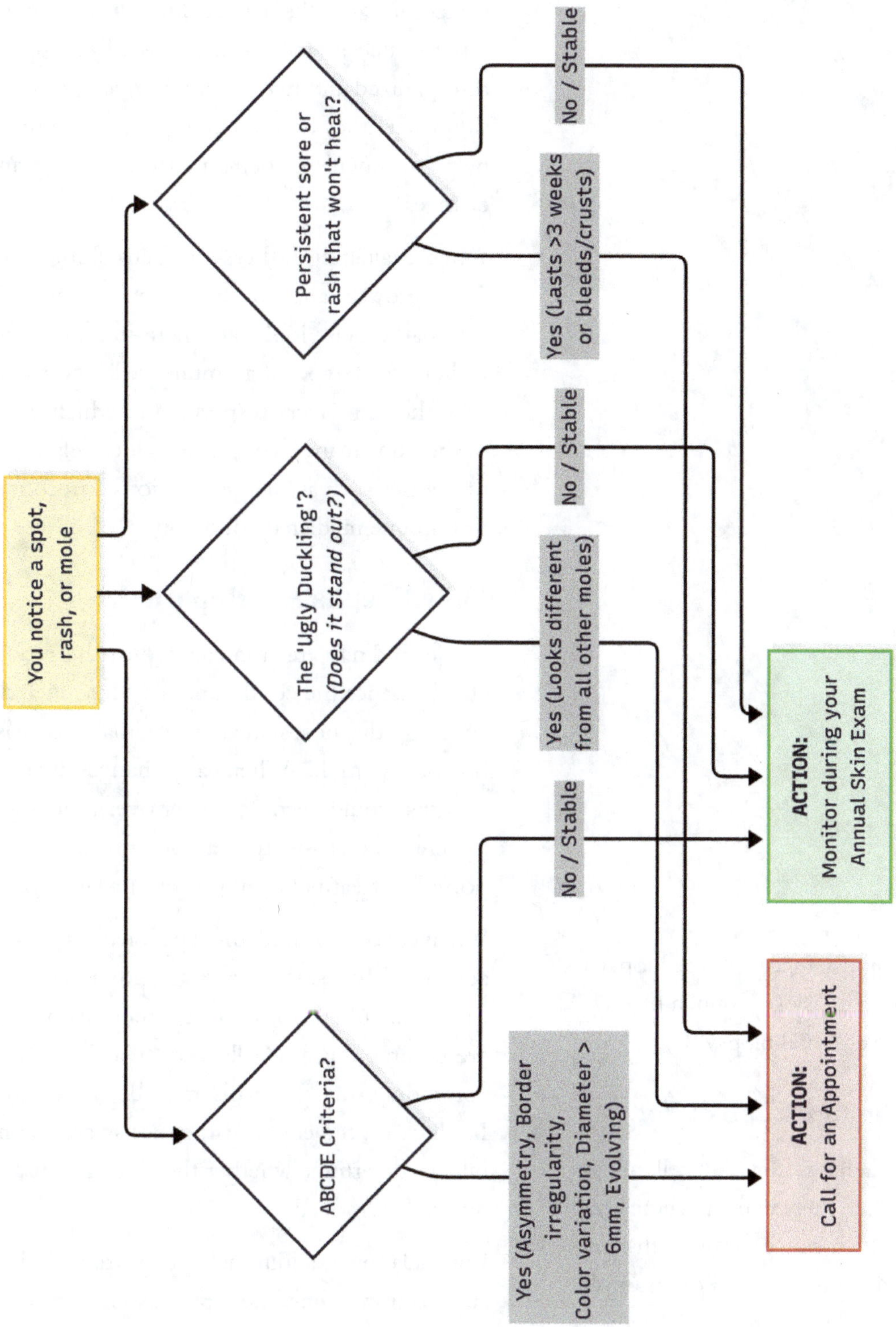
You notice a spot, rash, or mole
ABCDE Criteria?
Yes (Asymmetry, Border irregularity, Color variation, Diameter > 6mm, Evolving)
No / Stable
The 'Ugly Duckling'? (Does it stand out?)
Yes (Looks different from all other moles)
No / Stable
Persistent sore or rash that won't heal?
Yes (Lasts >3 weeks or bleeds/crusts)
No / Stable
ACTION: Call for an Appointment
ACTION: Monitor during your Annual Skin Exam

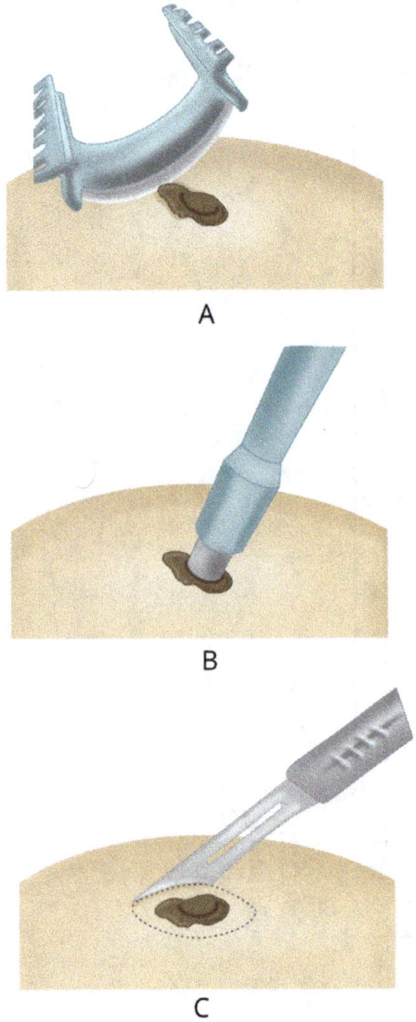

Figure 8: Skin biopsy types and the biopsy tools used: shave biopsy (A), punch biopsy (B), and excisional biopsy (C)

What the Pathologist Looks For

The pathologist examines how skin cells are arranged and whether they remain where they normally belong. Non-cancerous growths tend to be orderly and contained. For example, most harmless moles are symmetrical, balanced in shape, and confined to the expected layers of the skin.

Cancerous growths behave differently. In conditions such as melanoma, cells often appear disorganized and may extend into layers of the skin where they do not belong. These patterns help distinguish benign from malignant changes.

When evaluating rashes, the focus shifts away from growth and toward reaction patterns. The pathologist looks at where immune cells gather, what type of immune cells there are, how the skin layers respond, and which parts of the skin are involved. These clues help identify causes such as allergic reactions, infections, or immune mediated conditions.

How Results Are Reported

If the findings are non-cancerous, the report clearly names the condition. This may include common diagnoses such as eczema, psoriasis, or a benign mole. When early changes are present that could become cancer over time, such as actinic keratosis, they are identified and reported so treatment can prevent progression.

When cancer is found, the report names the exact type. Most skin cancers are either basal cell carcinoma or squamous cell carcinoma, which are common and usually very treatable. Less commonly, the diagnosis may be melanoma. In all cases, the edges of the biopsy are examined to determine whether the abnormal tissue was fully removed.

For melanoma, additional details are included, such as how deeply the tumor extends into the skin. This information is critical because it directly guides treatment decisions and follow up planning.

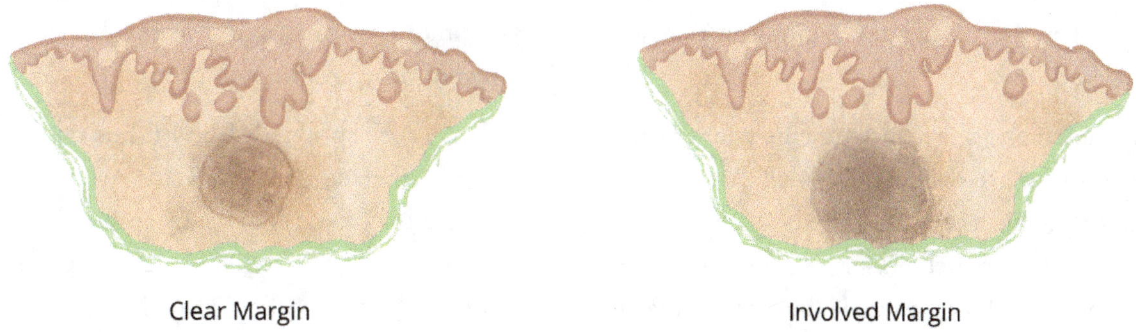

Figure 9. Examples of clear margin and positive margin (i.e. tumor present on edge of biopsy)

What Happens Next

When results are benign, many conditions require little or no treatment. Some rashes respond to creams or ointments. Others simply need time to resolve. Your clinician will explain whether any follow up is recommended or whether reassurance is all that is needed.

Occasionally, a biopsy may show that abnormal cells extend to the edge (margin) of the tissue sample. Even if the finding is non-cancerous, or represents an early-stage, low-risk condition, additional steps may be recommended to ensure the area is completely clear. This might include topical treatments or a minor follow-up procedure. These steps are typically straightforward and are performed primarily to reduce the risk of the condition returning.

When skin cancer is diagnosed, it is often caught at an early stage. Early cancers are typically treated with localized procedures that remove any remaining abnormal cells. These treatments are highly effective and are usually performed in an outpatient or office setting.

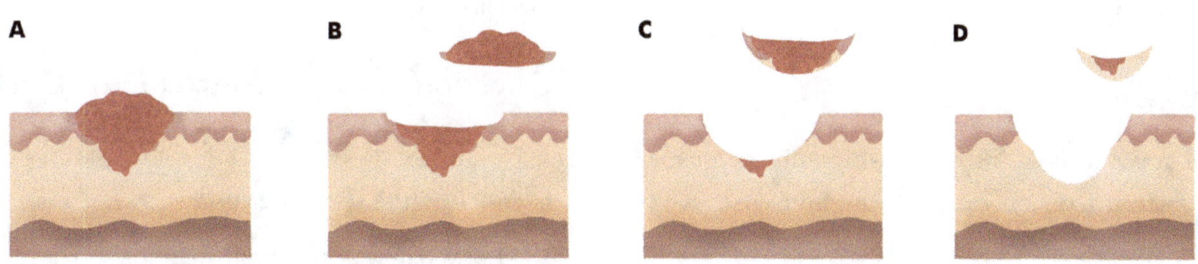

Figure 10. Moh's micrographic surgery explained (A: tumor; B: first stage removal; C: Second stage removal; D: last stage removal with clear margins)

Common Fears and Reassurances

Almost every patient I have ever spoken to about a skin biopsy worries first about the scar. I understand the worry. The skin is the only organ we see in the mirror, and a small white mark on your forearm is more visible than the entire silent landscape inside your abdomen.

But after years of signing out dermatopathology, I have come to think of the scar differently. It is the receipt for a question that got answered.

The punch and shave instruments your dermatologist uses are deliberately small. A four-millimeter punch leaves a mark about the size of the head of a pencil eraser; in most places on the body it fades into a pale line within a year. What does not fade is the diagnosis. Once I have looked at the slide and written down what those cells actually are, that question is closed. You and your dermatologist can move forward, build a routine of sunscreen and yearly checks, and stop wondering about the spot.

Peace of Mind and Prevention

Skin biopsies are performed when clinical examination including dermoscopic examination is not enough to diagnose a medical condition. The answer the biopsy returns is what lets your dermatologist stop estimating and start treating — or, just as often, stop watching a spot they were unsure about. Sunscreen, protective clothing, and a yearly skin check do more to prevent the next biopsy than anything else available.

Example

A rough, raised, ashy, dark-brown spot raised concern for skin cancer. The biopsy showed seborrheic keratosis, a very common and completely harmless growth that usually arises on a sun-damaged skin. No additional treatment was needed, and the result provided immediate peace of mind.

A flat, scaly patch on sun exposed skin was biopsied and diagnosed as actinic keratosis, an early change caused by long term sun damage. Because it is precancerous, topical treatment (commonly fluorouracil) was recommended to prevent progression over time.

A small dark spot with a bluish hue raised concern for melanoma. Under the microscope, it proved to be a blue nevus, a benign mole caused by pigment cells located deeper in the skin.

What This Means for You

A skin biopsy is usually quick and straightforward. The area is numbed, discomfort is minimal, and recovery is typically simple. Within days, the report explains exactly what was found and whether any further care is needed.

Most results lead to reassurance or straightforward treatment. Some findings require a small additional procedure to ensure complete removal. When skin cancer is identified, it is often caught early and treated effectively.

Most skin biopsies settle the question. A spot that looked ambiguous is named, and what comes next — observation, a cream, a small additional procedure — follows directly from that name.

Questions to Ask Your Doctor During a Follow-up Appointment

Understanding the Diagnosis

1. What was the final diagnosis? (Is it a growth, an inflammatory rash, or an infection?)
2. Was the diagnosis benign, atypical, or malignant?

3. If it is a rash, did the biopsy point to a specific cause, like an allergy or an immune response?

Understanding the Pathology Report

1. Were the margins clear? (if the entire area of concern was removed or if abnormal cells were found at the very edge of the sample.)
2. If it is skin cancer, how deep or thick was the growth? (This is especially important for melanoma results.)
3. Is there a copy of the pathology report I can have for my records?

Next Steps and Treatment

1. Do I need any further treatment or procedures?
2. If treatment is needed, what are my options? (e.g., creams, a minor surgical excision, or simple monitoring.)
3. How should I care for the biopsy site as it continues to heal?

Long-Term Prevention

1. Does this result increase my risk for other skin issues in the future?
2. How often should I come back for a full-body skin check?
3. Are there specific changes I should look for in my skin at home?

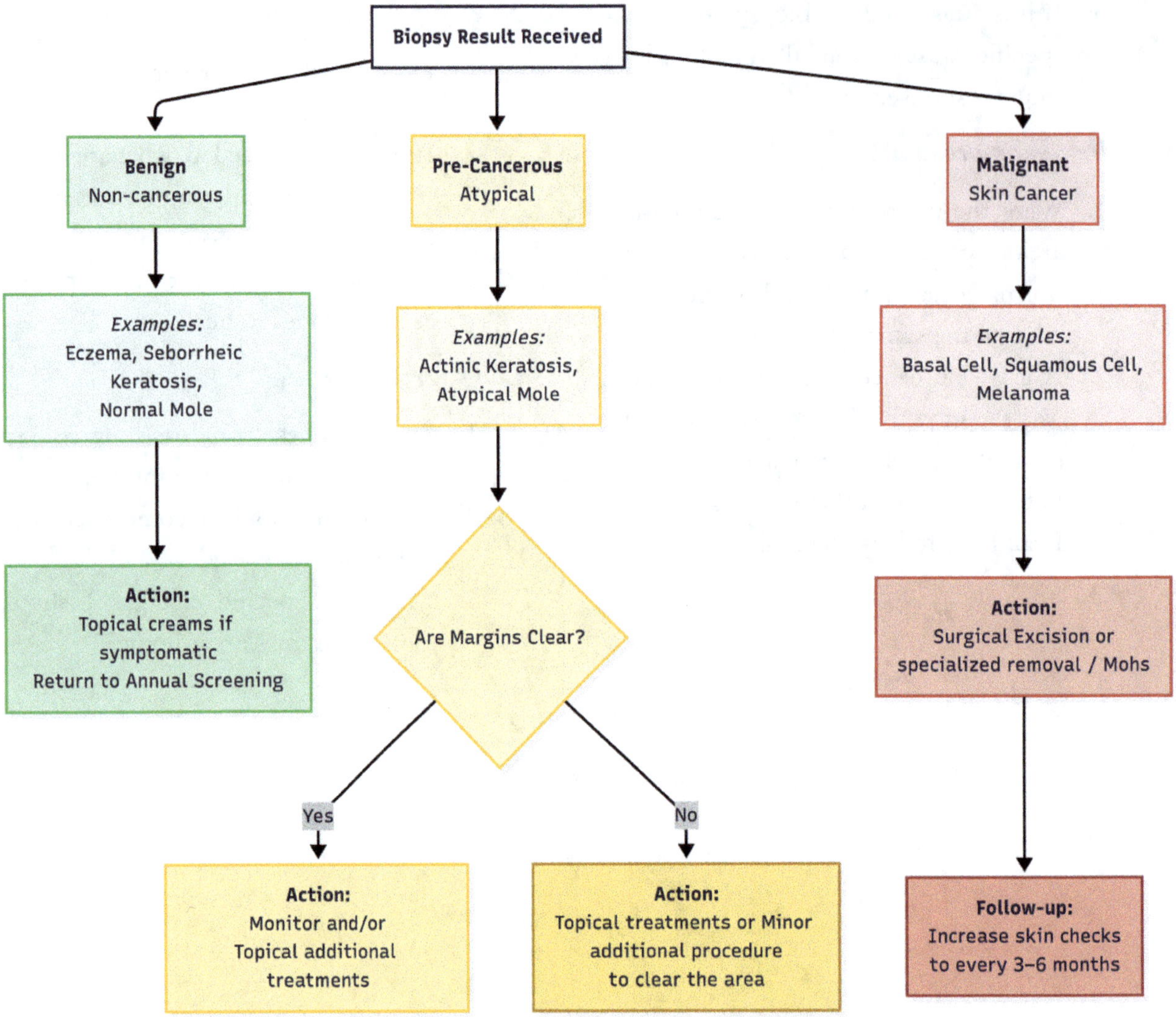

Recommended Skin Exam Protocol

Dermatologists work to identify skin problems, track biopsy results, and manage in a professional and organized way to protect long-term skin health. Modern electronic health record systems make this easy and possible.

Monthly Self-Exams

The American Academy of Dermatology recommends checking your own skin once a month. Use a full-length mirror and a hand mirror to check hard-to-see areas like your back and scalp. Look for the ABCDEs of moles:

Asymmetry: One half does not match the other.
Border: Edges are ragged, blurred, or irregular.
Color: The color is not uniform (shades of tan, brown, black, or even blue/red).
Diameter: The spot is larger than 6mm (about the size of a pencil eraser).
Evolving: The mole is changing in size, shape, or color.

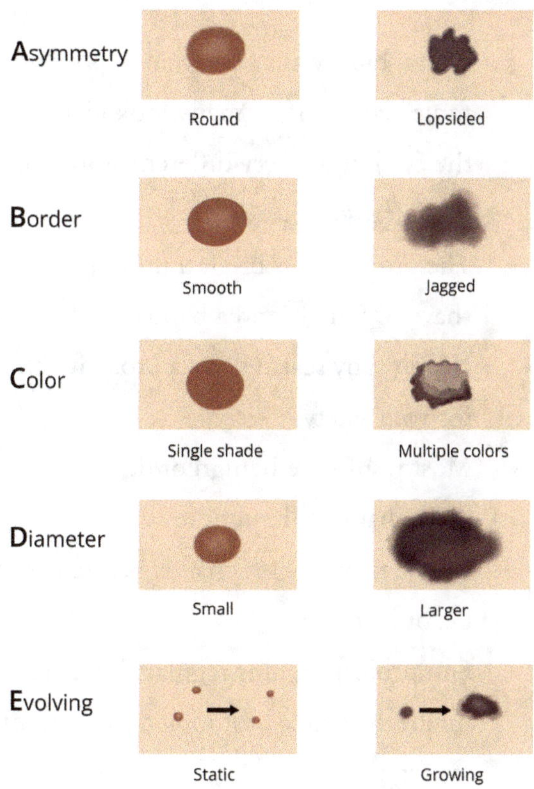

Figure 11. The ABCDE rule illustration.

The Ugly Duckling Sign

In addition to the ABCDEs, look for the Ugly Duckling. Most moles on your body will look similar to one another. A spot that looks, feels, or grows differently than all your other moles is a primary candidate for a biopsy.

Annual Professional Total Body Skin Exam (TBSE)

- For the general population, a professional head-to-toe exam by a dermatologist is recommended once a year.
- If you have a history of skin cancer, numerous moles (atypical nevus syndrome), or significant sun damage, your doctor may recommend exams every 3 to 6 months.
- During this exam, the clinician often uses a dermatoscope, a handheld magnifier with a polarized light, to see structures beneath the skin's surface that are invisible to the naked eye.

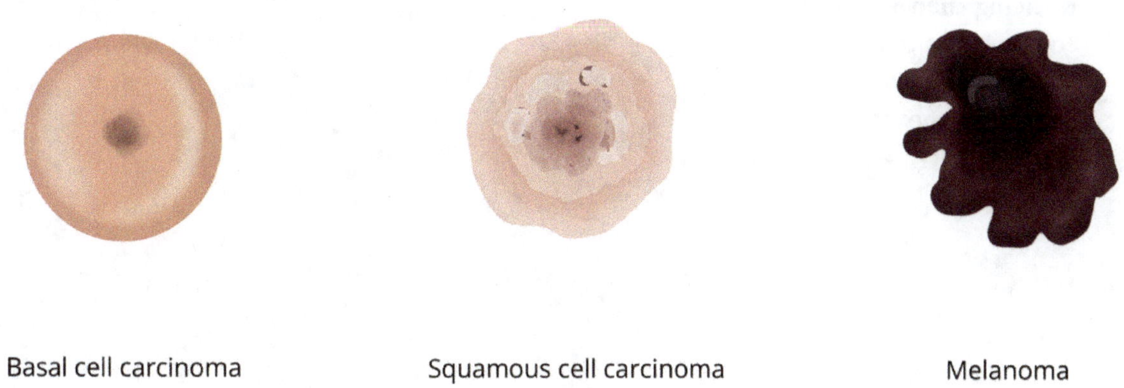

Figure 12. Visual examination appearance of different skin cancer types

Professional Baseline

If you have never had a skin exam, dermatologists recommend getting a baseline screening. This allows your doctor to document your existing moles, making it much easier to identify new or changing spots during future visits.

> **Author Tip: The 'Surface Clues' Secret**
>
> **What You See Matters:** Many skin conditions reveal themselves through subtle changes in texture – not just color.
>
> If the surface looks unusually shiny, rough, thickened, or finely wrinkled, these early shifts can point your doctor toward the right diagnosis.
>
> **Noticing changes early** often leads to faster answers and simpler treatments.

Quick Summary

- A skin biopsy answers what a spot, rash, or mole actually is — many look identical to the eye but tell very different stories under the microscope.
- The procedure is brief: numbing, a small shave or punch, and a bandage. Most heal cleanly; any scar reflects a proactive choice for your safety.
- Most results are benign or describe an early change (like actinic keratosis) that can be treated with creams before it ever becomes cancer.
- Sun protection plus regular skin checks remains the single best long-term prevention strategy.
- Use the ABCDE rule and the "ugly duckling" sign for monthly self-checks. Anyone with prior skin cancer or many atypical moles needs a professional exam every 3–6 months.

Chapter 10

Breast Core Needle Biopsy

From ambiguity to clarity

What It Is and Why It's Done

Modern breast imaging is excellent at detecting small or subtle changes. Mammograms, ultrasound, and MRI can reveal areas that look different from surrounding tissue, often long before they cause symptoms. However, imaging alone cannot always determine whether a finding is harmless, high risk, or cancerous.

When an area needs clarification, a breast core needle biopsy allows doctors to sample the exact spot seen on imaging which provides detailed information about the nature of the cells.

Today, the goal of a breast biopsy goes beyond answering the question of whether cancer is present. If the diagnosis is cancer, understanding its exact type and biological behavior is essential. This information allows treatment to be personalized, targeted, and not more aggressive than necessary.

How the Biopsy Is Performed

Before the biopsy begins, the skin and deeper tissues are numbed so discomfort is minimal. A hollow needle is then used to collect several small cylinders of tissue, called cores, from the area of concern.

The procedure is guided by imaging to ensure accuracy. Depending on the location of the finding, guidance may be provided by mammography, ultrasound, or MRI. This real time imaging allows the needle to be directed precisely to the abnormal area.

The biopsy itself is usually brief. A tiny metal marker may be placed at the biopsy site so the area can be identified again if needed for future imaging or surgery. Most people go home shortly afterward. Mild soreness or bruising is common for a few days, while serious complications are uncommon.

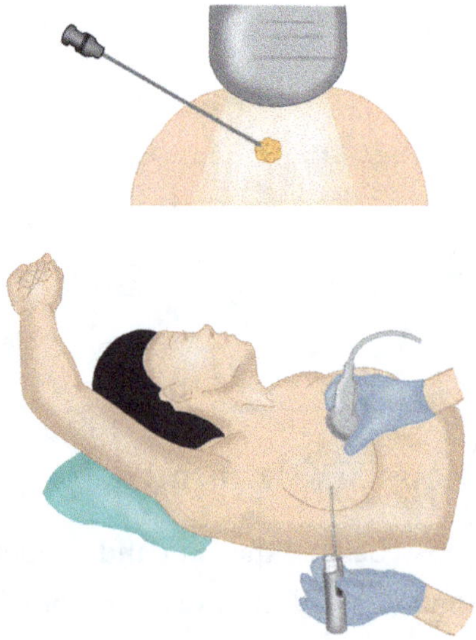

Figure 13. Ultrasound guided core needle biopsy of the breast

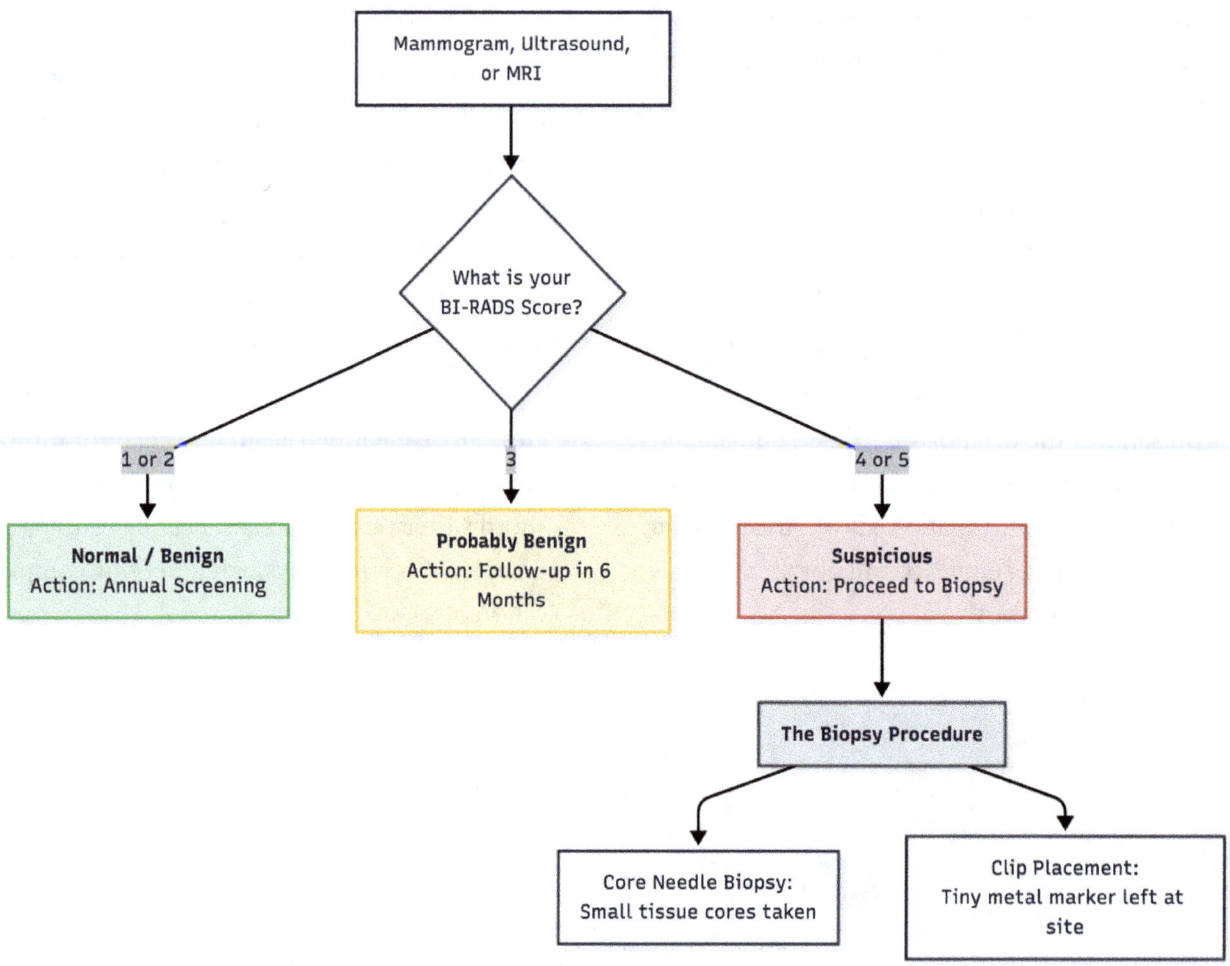

Decision Flow Why Am I Here?

What the Pathologist Looks For

Under the microscope, the pathologist determines whether the tissue represents a benign condition, a high risk or in situ process, or invasive cancer. Benign findings include common conditions such as fibroadenomas or fibrocystic changes. High risk changes or in situ lesions, such as ductal carcinoma in situ, are confined to their original structures and have not invaded surrounding tissue.

When invasive cancer is present, abnormal cells have moved beyond their normal boundaries. The pathologist identifies the specific type, such as invasive ductal or invasive lobular carcinoma, and evaluates how aggressive the cells appear. These features help predict behavior and guide treatment choices.

Some cores may contain calcifications, which are tiny calcium deposits that can be associated with conditions such as ductal carcinoma in situ, an early form of breast cancer confined to the milk ducts.

An important part of evaluation is correlation. The pathologist compares what is seen under the microscope with what the radiologist saw on imaging. This step confirms that the sampled tissue matches the targeted abnormality and helps ensure that the correct area was evaluated.

How Results Are Reported

Breast biopsy reports include both a diagnosis and biological features that guide therapy. These biologic features, often called biomarkers, act as keys that open or close certain treatment options.

Hormone receptors indicate whether the tumor is likely to respond to medications that block estrogen or progesterone. Another important marker identifies whether targeted therapies aimed at a specific growth pathway may be effective. Together, these results help determine whether hormone therapy, targeted therapy, chemotherapy, or a combination is most appropriate.

What Happens Next

When the biopsy shows benign changes, the usual next step is imaging follow up rather than treatment. Many findings simply return to routine surveillance.

If precancerous or cancerous changes are identified, the biopsy result decides what comes next. Some patients benefit from surgery as the first step. Others may begin with medication to shrink or control the tumor before surgery. The approach is shaped by the tumor's biology as well as the patient's preferences and overall health.

Treatment planning is typically done by a multidisciplinary team that includes radiologists, surgeons, oncologists, and pathologists, all working from the same shared information.

Common Fears and Reassurances

The waiting is often the hardest part. I have signed out breast biopsies most weeks of my career, and I know the shape of those few days from the patient's side: the mammogram callback, the targeted ultrasound, the radiologist's careful phrasing, the appointment for cores, then silence. I want to tell you what those days look like from my side, because the silence is not empty.

Once your samples arrive in the lab, they are processed overnight, cut onto slides the next morning, and stained. By the time I see them, the radiologist's image is already pulled up beside me. I am comparing the calcifications they targeted with what is actually in the tissue. I am asking, before anything else, did we sample the right thing? Roughly four out of five breast biopsies will come back benign. Of the ones that do show cancer, most are detected at a stage where the treatment is tailored, often modest, and very effective. The numbers were not always this kind. They are this kind now because the imaging is good, the cores are well placed, and the slides reach pathologists who have read tens of thousands of them.

Example

Tiny calcifications were detected on a routine screening mammogram. A core needle biopsy revealed ductal carcinoma in situ that was sensitive to hormone receptor blocking medication. Breast conserving surgery followed by targeted hormone therapy provided excellent disease control, without the need for chemotherapy.

Early detection and precise characterization allowed treatment to be effective without being excessive.

What This Means for You

A breast core needle biopsy provides more than a diagnosis. It provides a roadmap. A few carefully targeted samples can reveal whether a finding is benign, precancerous, or invasive cancer, as well as which treatments are most likely to help.

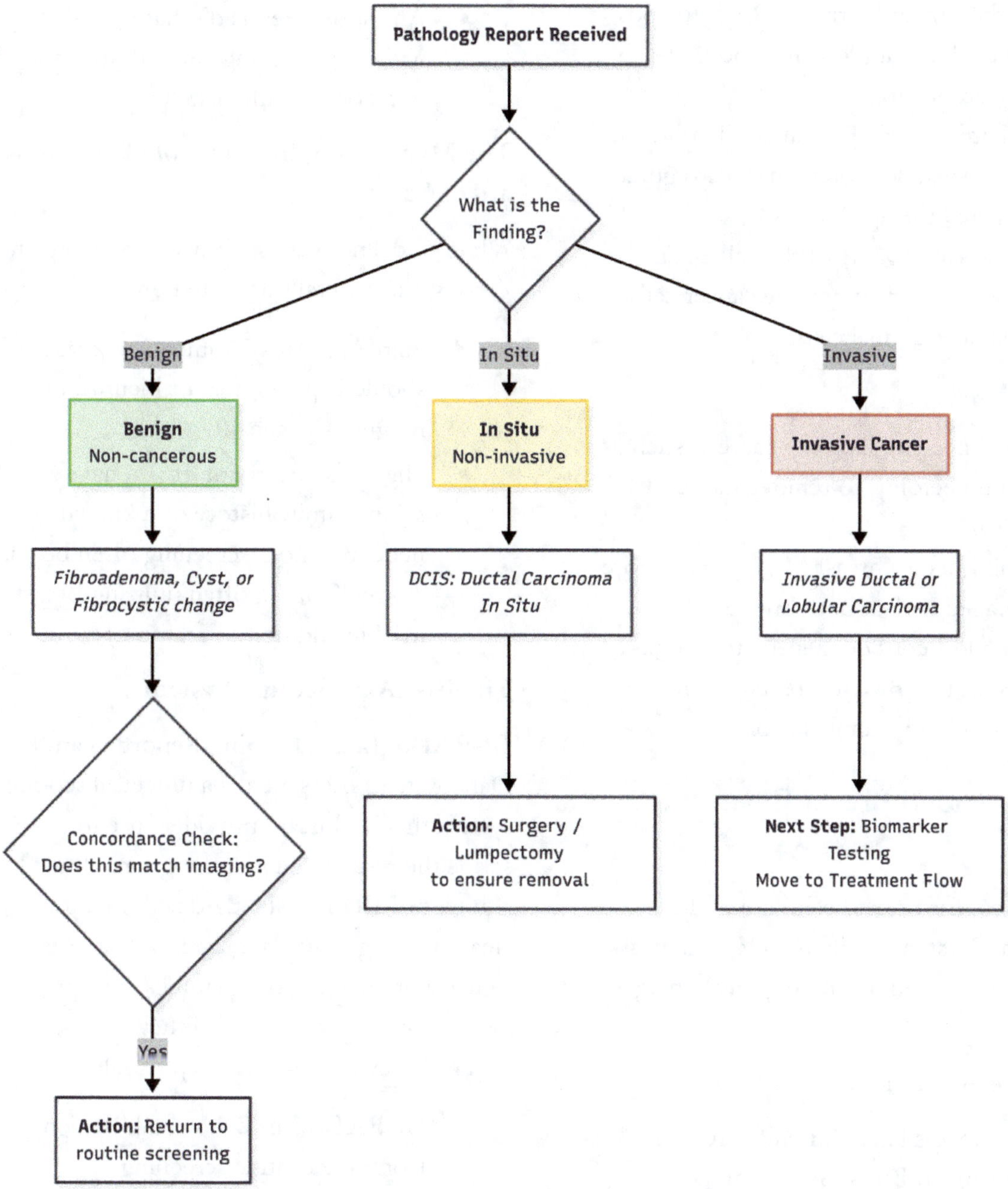

Questions to Ask Your Doctor During a Follow-up Appointment

On the Results and Findings

1. What was the specific diagnosis? (e.g., Was it a Fibroadenoma, a Cyst, Ductal Carcinoma In Situ (DCIS), or Invasive Ductal Carcinoma?)
2. If it is non-cancerous, does it increase my future risk? (Some benign findings, like atypical ductal hyperplasia, require closer monitoring than others.)
3. Was the biopsy concordant? (This is asking if the pathology result matches what was seen on the imaging.)

For Cancerous Results

1. Is the cancer Hormone Receptor-positive? (Does it grow in response to Estrogen or Progesterone?)
2. What is the HER2 status? (This identifies a specific protein that helps guide targeted therapy.)
3. What is the grade of the cells? (This describes how much the cancer cells look like normal cells.)

On Next Steps

1. Do I need a follow-up surgery, such as a lumpectomy, to remove the rest of the area?
2. Will I need a breast MRI to get a more detailed look at both breasts?
3. Should I consider genetic testing (like BRCA1 or BRCA2) based on these results and my family history?

Recommended Breast Exam Protocol

The protocol for breast health is a multi-layered defense system involving self-awareness, professional evaluation, and high-tech imaging.

Breast Self-Awareness

Modern protocols have shifted from rigid monthly exams to Breast Self-Awareness. This means knowing what is normal for your breasts so you can spot changes:

- Check in the mirror for skin dimpling, nipple inversion, or redness.
- Be aware of new lumps, thickening, or knots that don't go away after your menstrual cycle.
- Any spontaneous discharge (leaking without squeezing) should be reported to a doctor immediately.

The Mammography Protocol (The standard of Care)

While guidelines vary slightly between organizations, the generally accepted protocol is:

- Start Age: Most women at average risk should begin annual or biennial mammograms at age 40.
- High-Risk Protocol: If you have a strong family history or a known genetic mutation, screening often begins at age 25 or 30, often utilizing Breast MRI in addition to mammograms.

The BI-RADS Scoring System

BI-RADS (Breast Imaging-Reporting and Data System) is essentially a universal scoring system that healthcare providers use to describe the results of a mammogram, ultrasound, or **MRI** in a standardized way. Instead of using vague language, radiologists assign a score from 0 to 6 that tells your provider exactly how concerned they are about a finding and what the next step should be.

- **BI-RADS 1 or 2**: Normal/Benign. Continue routine screening.
- **BI-RADS 3**: Probably benign. Protocol dictates a short-interval follow-up (usually in 6 months).
- **BI-RADS 4 or 5**: Suspicious. Protocol dictates a biopsy is necessary.
- **BI-RADS 6**: Known cancer, biopsy proven

The Tissue Clip

During most breast biopsies, the clinician

performing the biopsy will place a tiny metal clip (smaller than a grain of rice) at the site. This is a universal protocol that allows future mammograms to identify exactly where the biopsy was taken, allowing tracking of that specific for years to come.

Too small to feel, but big enough for a mammogram to see.

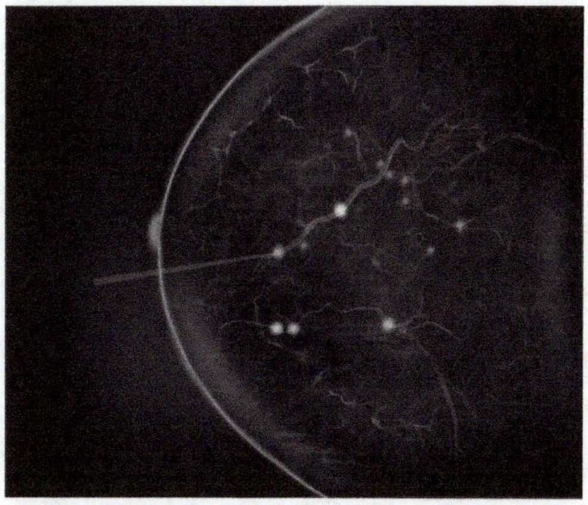

Figure 14. Mammogram showing white spots of calcifications

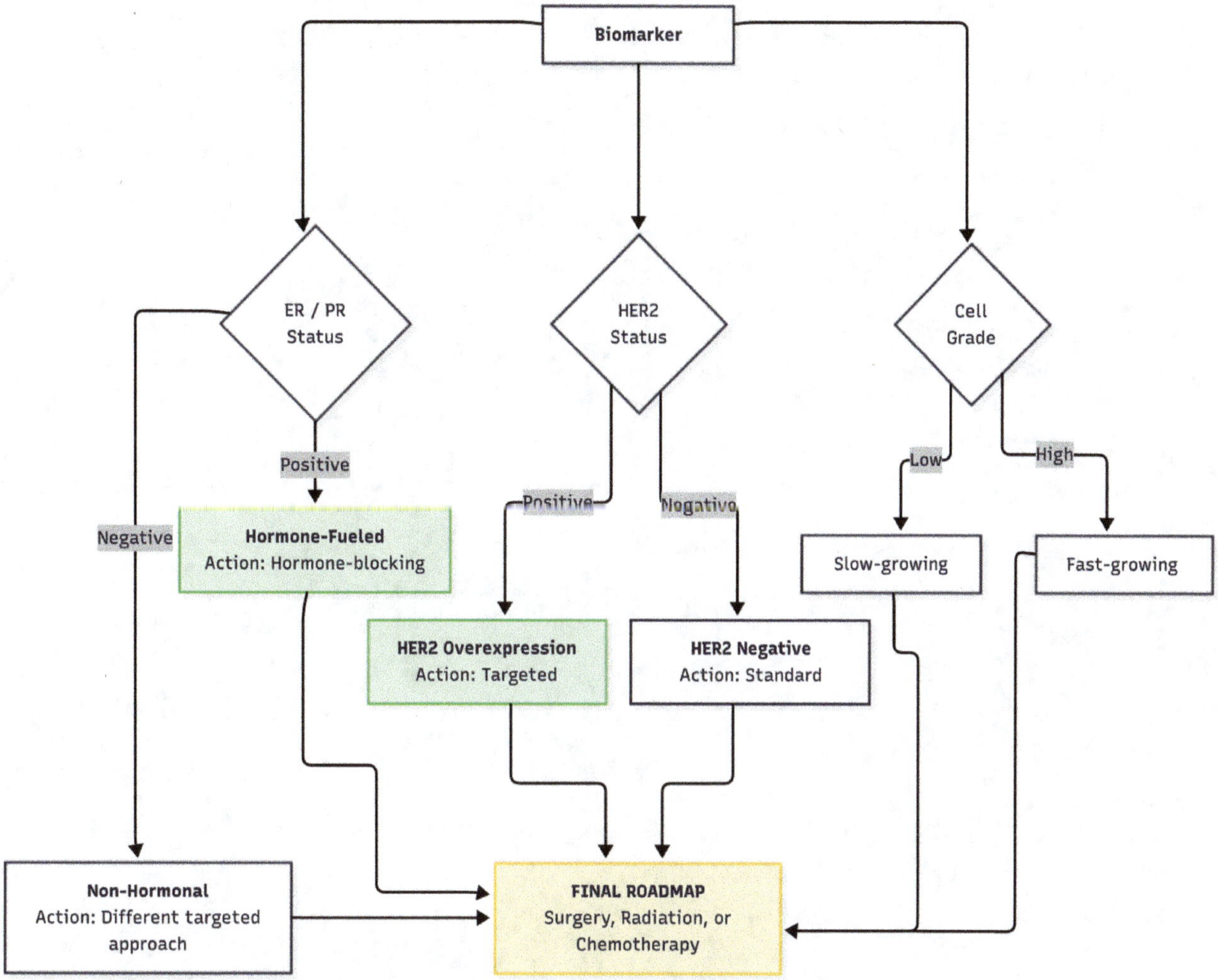

The Biomarker Roadmap to Treatment

Quick Summary

- A core needle biopsy uses imaging guidance (mammogram, ultrasound, or MRI) to sample exactly the spot of concern, providing certainty that imaging alone cannot.
- The biopsy answers both whether the finding is cancer and, if so, the biological features (hormone receptors, HER2) that determine which treatments will work.
- A tiny tissue marker (clip) is placed at the biopsy site so the area can be tracked or located again on future mammograms.
- About 80% of breast biopsies return benign results — the test most often rules out cancer rather than confirming it.
- Modern care is multidisciplinary and personalized. Treatment depends as much on the tumor's biology as on its size, so two patients with the same diagnosis may follow very different plans.

Chapter 11

Endometrial Biopsy

Making Sense of Abnormal Uterine Bleeding

What It Is and Why It's Done

An endometrial biopsy examines a small sample of the lining of the uterus, called the endometrium. It is most often performed to explain unexpected uterine bleeding, especially bleeding after menopause, irregular bleeding patterns, or a thickened uterine lining seen on ultrasound.

The endometrium is a hormonally responsive tissue. Its appearance normally changes over the course of the menstrual cycle and shifts again after menopause. For this reason, what is considered normal depends strongly on age, menstrual status, and hormone exposure among others. Imaging can show thickness, but it cannot determine whether the tissue itself is normal, overgrown, or abnormal at a cellular level.

Biopsy unmasks the truth beneath by allowing direct examination of the lining itself. It distinguishes normal hormone related changes from benign growths, precancerous conditions, or cancer, guiding decisions with far greater precision.

How the Biopsy Is Performed

An endometrial biopsy is usually performed in the office and typically does not require anesthesia. A thin, flexible tube, often called a Pipelle, is gently passed through the cervix into the uterus. Light suction is used to collect a small portion of the lining.

The procedure is brief and usually lasts only a few minutes. Some people experience short lived cramping during or shortly after the biopsy, similar to menstrual cramps. This discomfort generally resolves quickly, and most patients are able to return to normal activities the same day.

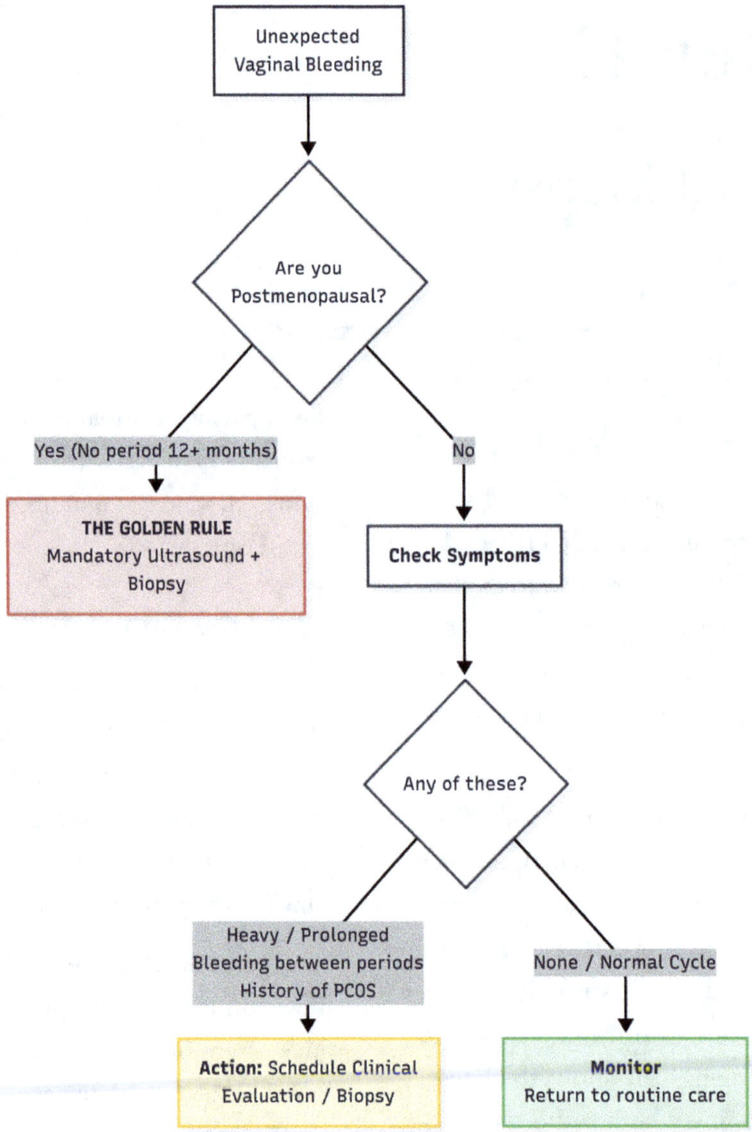

What the Pathologist Looks For

The first step is assessing whether enough endometrial tissue is present to make a reliable diagnosis. Adequacy is especially important because the endometrial lining naturally becomes thin at certain times of life, particularly after menopause.

After adequacy is confirmed, the tissue is examined for normal hormonal patterns, benign growths such as polyps, or hyperplasia, which refers to overgrowth of the lining. The cells are also evaluated for atypia, meaning abnormal features that indicate a higher risk of progression to cancer.

Under the microscope, the pathologist first determines whether the endometrium shows a normal hormonal pattern appropriate for the patient's age and clinical history. This includes comparing gland shape, spacing, and overall architecture with what would be expected for that life stage.

Attention is then given to identifying areas of crowding or excess growth. A key diagnosis the pathologist looks for is Endometrial Intraepithelial Neoplasia, often abbreviated as EIN and also known as atypical hyperplasia. This condition represents a true precancerous change that warrants treatment.

If abnormal cells have extended beyond the surface lining and invaded deeper, the diagnosis is endometrial carcinoma. This is the most common cancer of the uterus and one that is often highly treatable when detected early.

How Results Are Reported

The report links each diagnosis to a clear management path. Common terms you may see include descriptions of normal hormone-related patterns, benign polyps, hyperplasia with or without atypia, and endometrial carcinoma.

Each diagnosis carries a distinct clinical meaning. Benign polyps are common and often easily managed. Hyperplasia signals overgrowth with varying levels of cancer risk, depending on whether atypia is present. Cancer diagnoses prompt timely referral for staging and treatment planning.

The goal of the report is to guide the next step with accuracy.

What Happens Next

When results show normal or benign findings, management may involve observation, hormone adjustment, or simple treatment. In many cases, reassurance and monitoring are all that is needed.

If atypical hyperplasia or EIN is identified, a more proactive plan is recommended to prevent progression to cancer. Treatment decisions are individualized based on age, symptoms, and overall health.

When endometrial cancer is diagnosed, care moves promptly to staging and treatment planning. When detected early, outcomes are often excellent, and many patients are cured with timely intervention.

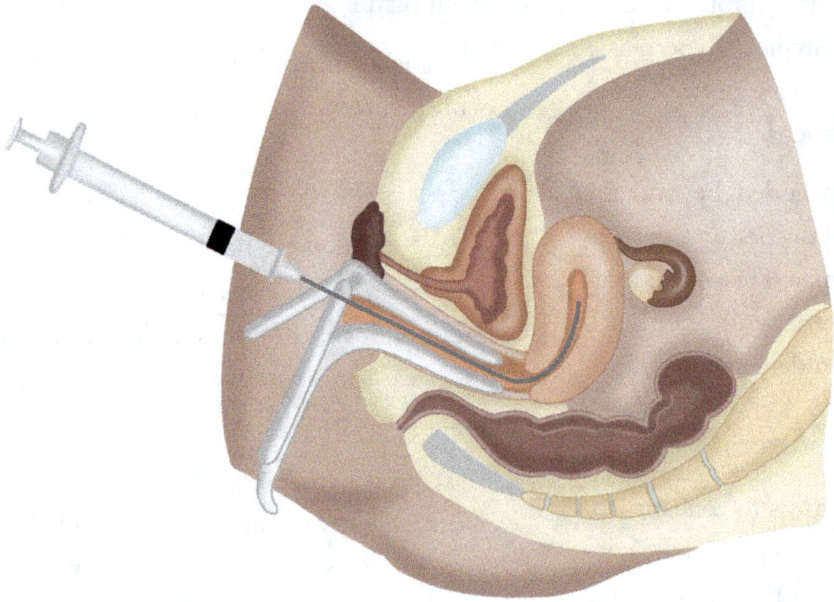

Figure 15. Endometrial biopsy using pipelle

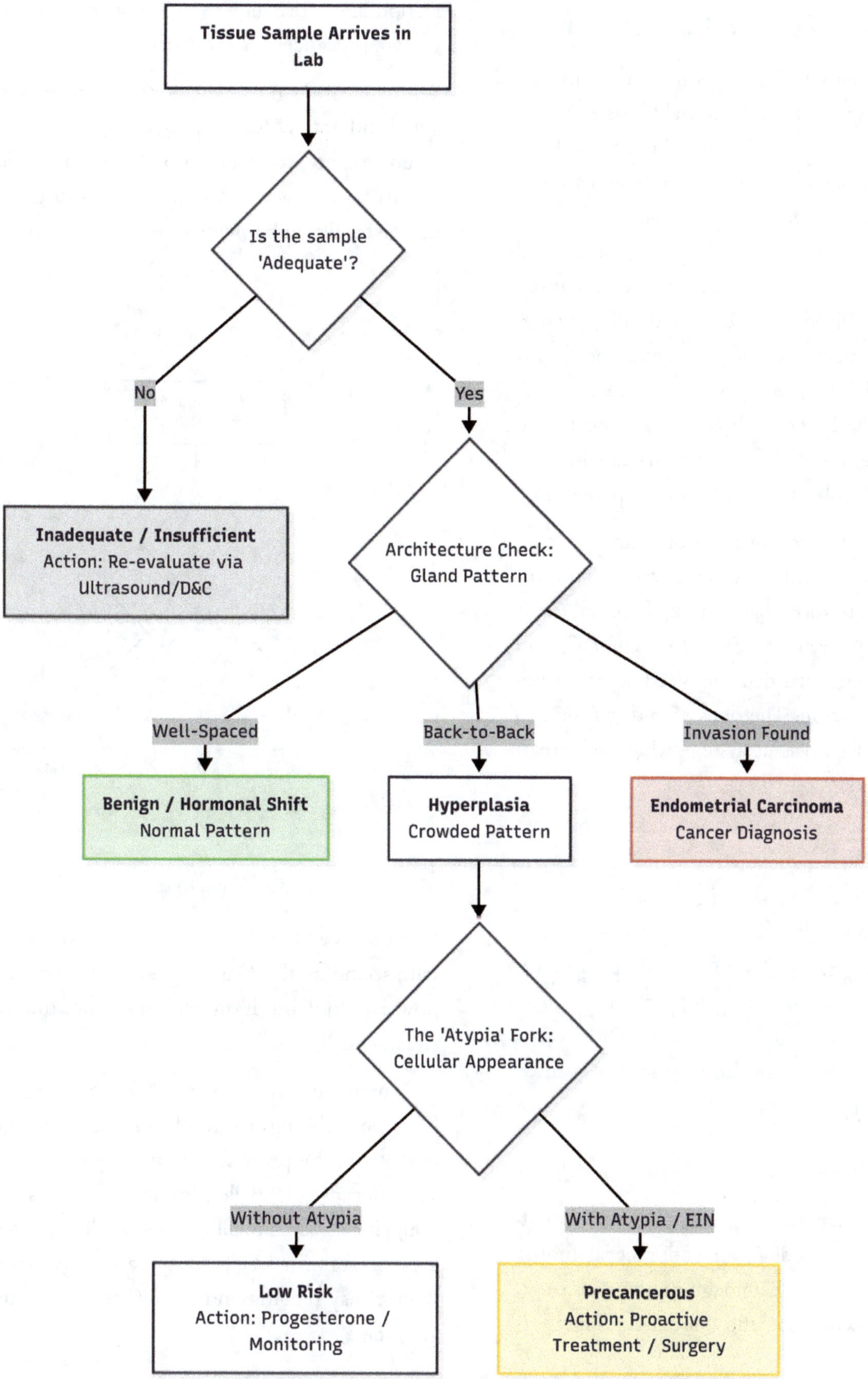
Tissue Sample Arrives in Lab
Is the sample 'Adequate'?
No
Yes
Inadequate / Insufficient
Action: Re-evaluate via Ultrasound/D&C
Architecture Check: Gland Pattern
Well-Spaced
Back-to-Back
Invasion Found
Benign / Hormonal Shift
Normal Pattern
Hyperplasia
Crowded Pattern
Endometrial Carcinoma
Cancer Diagnosis
The 'Atypia' Fork: Cellular Appearance
Without Atypia
With Atypia / EIN
Low Risk
Action: Progesterone / Monitoring
Precancerous
Action: Proactive Treatment / Surgery

Common Fears and Reassurances

Postmenopausal bleeding is the symptom that brings most of my endometrial biopsies to the lab, and I want to be honest about what I see when those slides arrive. Most of them are not cancer. Many show a benign polyp, or a thinned lining responding to hormonal changes, or a focal area of overgrowth that explains the bleeding without indicating malignancy. A smaller number show endometrial intraepithelial neoplasia, which is treatable. A smaller number still show frank cancer, and even there, the disease is typically caught early because the bleeding itself sent the patient in.

The biopsy is a few minutes of cramping in an office visit. The information it returns is the answer to a question that, left unanswered, tends to grow louder every week. Most women I read for go on to learn that the bleeding had a benign explanation. The ones who don't tend to get their diagnosis at a stage where the treatment works.

Example

A postmenopausal patient developed new vaginal bleeding and underwent an endometrial biopsy. The sample showed Endometrial Intraepithelial Neoplasia, a precancerous change. Because the condition was identified early, treatment was straightforward and prevented the development of invasive cancer.

What This Means for You

If you are experiencing unexplained or postmenopausal bleeding, an endometrial biopsy provides answers that imaging alone cannot. It clarifies whether the uterine lining is responding normally to hormones, is overgrown, precancerous, or cancerous.

With a clear diagnosis, next steps become targeted and timely. Rather than living with worry or uncertainty, you walk into the next appointment knowing what you have, and your gynecologist walks in knowing exactly what to treat.

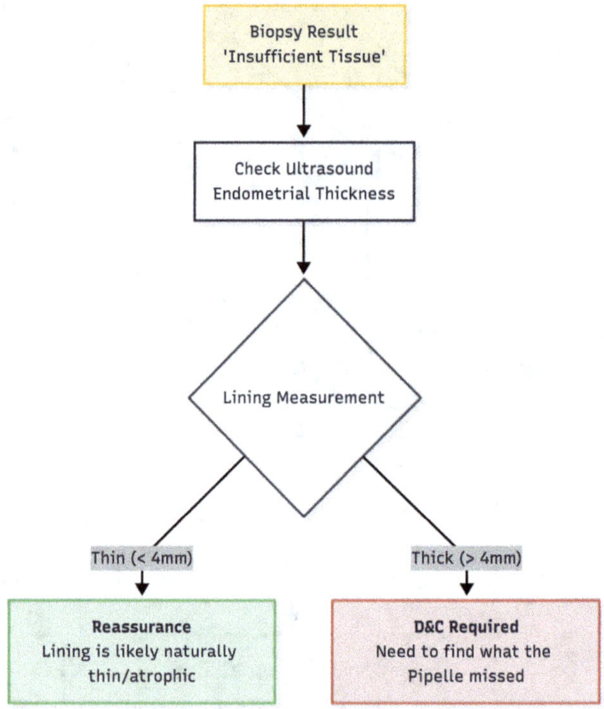

The Safety Net Logic

In the above Flowchart, it is helpful to think of Ultrasound as the Gatekeeper. A biopsy is a powerful tool, but it only tells us about the tissue it actually touches.

If your ultrasound shows a thick or irregular lining, but the biopsy result returns as benign or normal, the protocol often triggers a safety net. Because a Pipelle sample is a blind sampling, it can occasionally miss a small, localized area of abnormal cells. In these cases, your doctor may recommend a D&C (Dilation and Curettage).

Questions to Ask Your Doctor During a Follow-up Appointment

Understanding the Pathology Results

1. If hyperplasia was found, was it with atypia or without atypia? (Atypia refers to abnormal-looking cells and significantly changes the treatment plan.)
2. Were there any signs of polyps or fibroids that the biopsy might have detected?
3. Did the biopsy show enough tissue for a definitive answer? (Sometimes insufficient sample is reported if the lining was very thin.)

Determining the Cause

1. Does this result explain my abnormal bleeding?
2. Is this change related to a hormonal imbalance (like an estrogen/progesterone shift)?
3. Could my medications including HRT (if you're on Hormone Replacement Therapy) be influencing these results?

Next Steps & Treatment

1. If the result is benign but the bleeding continues, what is the next step?
2. Are there hormonal treatments that can help manage these findings?

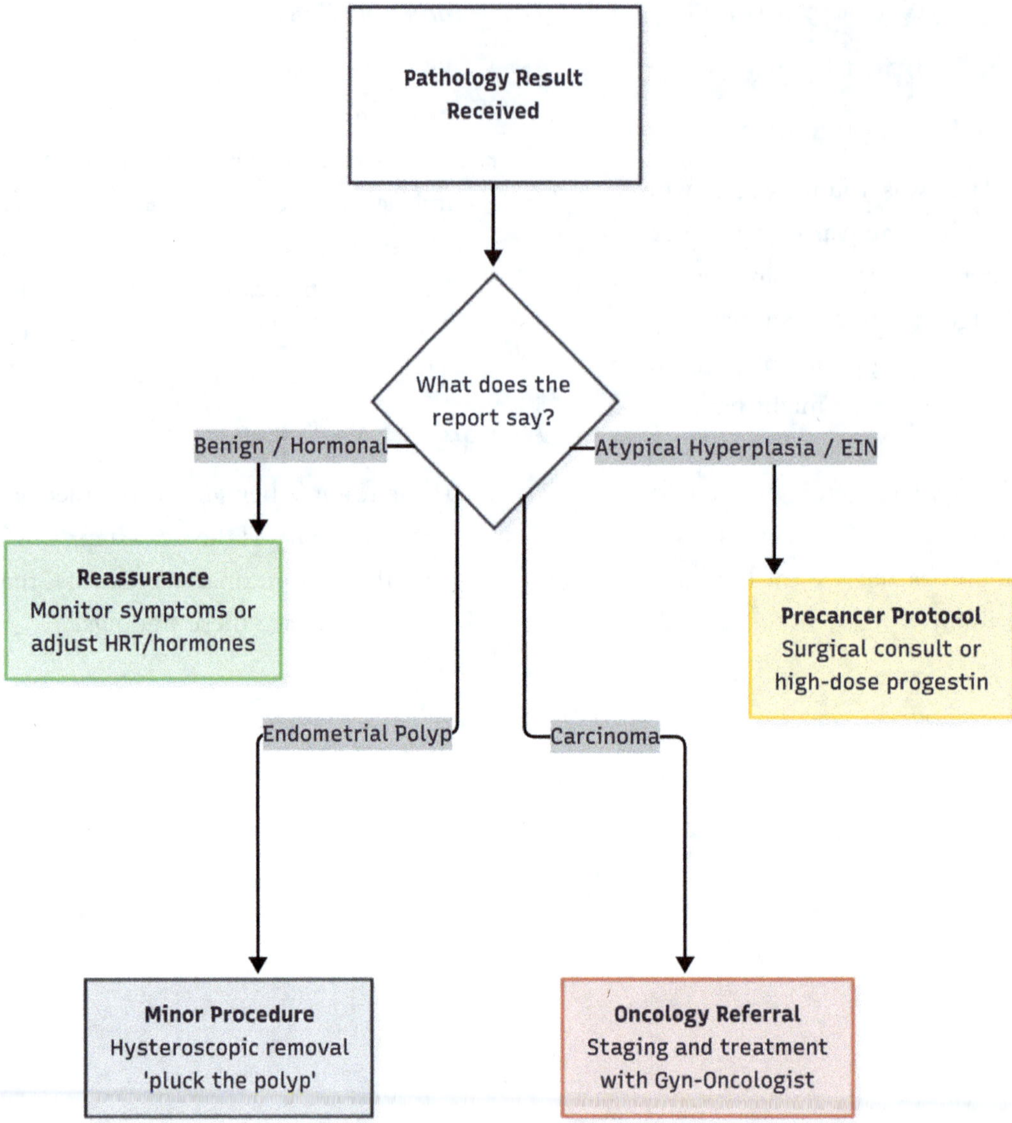

Recommended Endometrial Exam Protocol

Endometrial sampling is typically symptom-driven and usually not performed on a fixed schedule for everyone. However, there are universally accepted triggers for this protocol.

The Postmenopausal Standard

- Any vaginal bleeding after menopause (defined as 12 consecutive months without a period) is considered abnormal and must be evaluated.
- Often, a transvaginal ultrasound is the first step. If the endometrial thickness is greater than 4mm, a biopsy is usually the mandatory next step to rule out cancer.

The Abnormal Uterine Bleeding (AUB) Protocol

For those who have not reached menopause, a biopsy is recommended if you experience:

- Heavy or prolonged periods that interfere with daily life.
- Bleeding between periods (intermenstrual bleeding).
- Irregular cycles associated with conditions like PCOS (Polycystic Ovary Syndrome), which can lead to a buildup of the uterine lining.

High-Risk Surveillance

Certain individuals require more frequent monitoring regardless of symptoms:

- Lynch Syndrome: Patients with this genetic condition have a significantly higher risk of uterine cancer and often begin annual endometrial biopsies starting between ages 30 and 35.
- Tamoxifen Use: Patients taking Tamoxifen (for breast cancer) are monitored closely for any spotting, as the medication can occasionally cause the uterine lining to thicken.
- Unopposed Estrogen: If a patient is taking estrogen without progesterone, the protocol requires regular checks to ensure the lining isn't becoming overgrown (hyperplasia).

The Insufficient Sample Follow-up

If a biopsy comes back with insufficient tissue, the protocol dictates that the clinician must correlate this with an ultrasound. If the lining looks thick on the ultrasound but the biopsy was empty, a D&C (Dilation and Curettage) may be required to get a more thorough sample.

> 💡 **Author Tip: The 'Blind' Sample**
>
> **A Note on Accuracy:** An endometrial biopsy is a 'blind' procedure, meaning the doctor is not using a camera to see exactly where the sample is taken.
>
> It is very accurate for conditions that affect the whole lining, but it can occasionally miss a small, isolated polyp.
>
> This is why we always compare your biopsy results with your ultrasound 'picture'—if the two don't match, we keep looking.

Quick Summary

- An endometrial biopsy samples the uterine lining to explain abnormal bleeding — especially any bleeding after menopause, which always needs evaluation.
- The procedure is brief and done in the office without anesthesia. Cramping is common but usually short-lived.
- Imaging shows lining thickness but cannot reveal whether tissue is normal, overgrown, precancerous, or cancerous. Only the biopsy can.

- The key precancerous diagnosis is EIN (also called atypical hyperplasia). Identifying it allows treatment before invasive cancer develops.
- If imaging looks suspicious but the biopsy returns benign, a D&C may be needed because the office sample can miss small focal areas.

Chapter 12

Prostate Needle Biopsy

Clarity Without Overtreatment

What It Is and Why It's Done

A prostate needle biopsy is most often recommended after a rising PSA level, a concerning PSA trend over time, or a suspicious finding on prostate imaging such as MRI. It is important to understand that PSA is not a cancer specific test. Levels can rise for many reasons, including benign prostate enlargement, inflammation, infection, or prostate cancer.

Equally important, not all prostate cancers behave the same way. Some grow very slowly and may never cause symptoms or shorten life. Others are more aggressive and benefit from timely treatment. The purpose of a prostate biopsy is double pronged. (a) to confirm whether the finding is cancer; (b) if so, to determine how it is likely to behave.

This distinction allows care to be appropriate. Treatment can be active when necessary and conservative when it is safe.

How the Biopsy Is Performed

The biopsy is typically performed using local anesthesia and ultrasound guidance. With the guidance image in place, the urologist uses a thin needle to obtain multiple small tissue samples, called cores, from different regions of the prostate. Sampling several areas improves accuracy and ensures a representative evaluation.

If MRI has identified a specific area of concern, targeted samples may be taken from that location as well. These MRI guided cores increase precision, particularly for small or hard to reach lesions.

The procedure is usually done on an outpatient basis. Most men go home the same day and experience mild soreness, along with temporary urinary or rectal discomfort that resolves over a short time.

Different Biopsy Approaches

There are two main pathways used to reach the prostate. Transperineal and transrectal. Both are designed to obtain accurate samples, and the choice depends on anatomy, risk factors, and expertise.

In the transrectal approach, the needle passes through the wall of the rectum into the prostate under ultrasound guidance. This method is widely used and efficient. Because the needle crosses the rectal wall, antibiotics are given to reduce infection risk. Most men tolerate the procedure well, though a small risk of infection remains.

In the transperineal approach, the needle passes through the skin between the scrotum and anus rather than through the rectum. This route significantly lowers infection risk and allows better sampling of some regions of the prostate, especially the front portion. It may be done with local anesthesia or light sedation and is increasingly used in modern practice.

Regardless of the route, what matters most is the quality and accuracy of sampling. Both methods can be combined with MRI targeted biopsy to improve diagnostic precision.

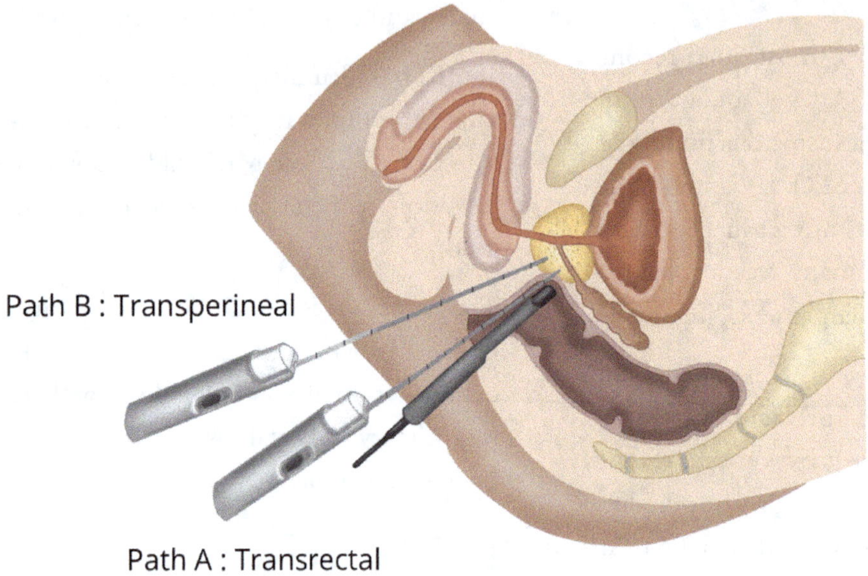

Figure 16. Transrectal and transperineal biopsy of the prostate

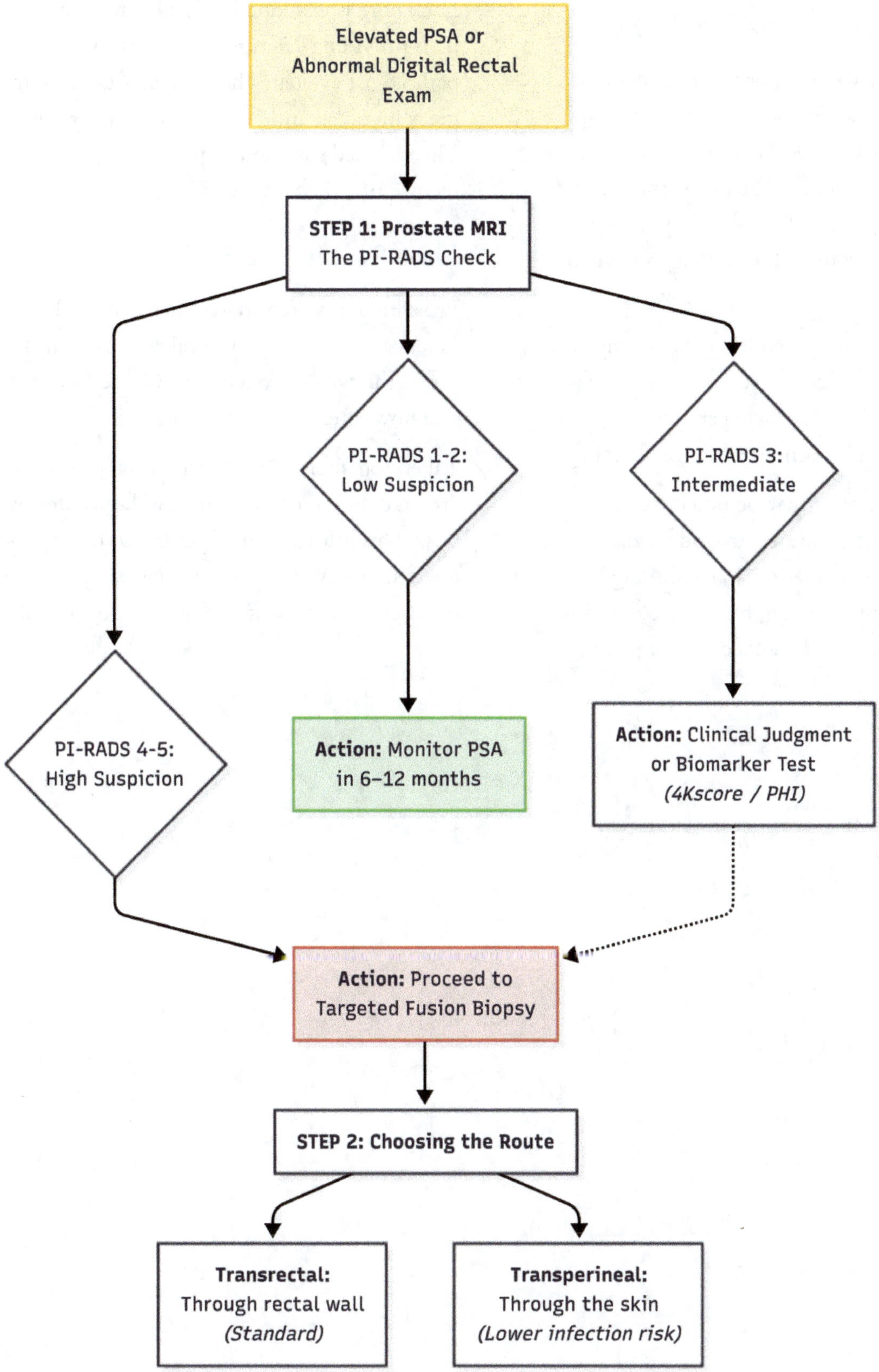

Elevated PSA or Abnormal Digital Rectal Exam
STEP 1: Prostate MRI
The PI-RADS Check
PI-RADS 1-2: Low Suspicion
PI-RADS 3: Intermediate
PI-RADS 4-5: High Suspicion
Action: Monitor PSA in 6–12 months
Action: Clinical Judgment or Biomarker Test (4Kscore / PHI)
Action: Proceed to Targeted Fusion Biopsy
STEP 2: Choosing the Route
Transrectal: Through rectal wall (Standard)
Transperineal: Through the skin (Lower infection risk)

What the Pathologist Looks For

Under the microscope, prostate cancer is graded using the Gleason system. This system evaluates how closely the cancer resembles normal prostate tissue and summarizes those findings into a Grade Group, ranging from Grade Group 1, the least aggressive, to Grade Group 5, the most aggressive.

Lower grade cancers tend to grow slowly and are often well suited for conservative management. Higher grade cancers are more likely to grow, spread, and benefit from treatment.

Additional features may be noted, such as cancer involving the area around small nerves, called perineural invasion. This finding helps with treatment planning, but by itself does not mean the cancer is advanced or dangerous.

Each core is examined individually. Rather than providing a simple yes or no answer, the pathologist evaluates how much of each sample is involved and how the cells are arranged. This detailed assessment provides a clearer picture of risk and behavior.

How Results Are Reported

Prostate biopsy reports are designed to be practical and clear. A typical result might describe the type of cancer, the Grade Group, and how much of a given core is involved.

Taken together, these details convey how aggressive the cancer appears and how extensive it is. This information is central to determining whether Active Surveillance is appropriate or whether treatment should be considered.

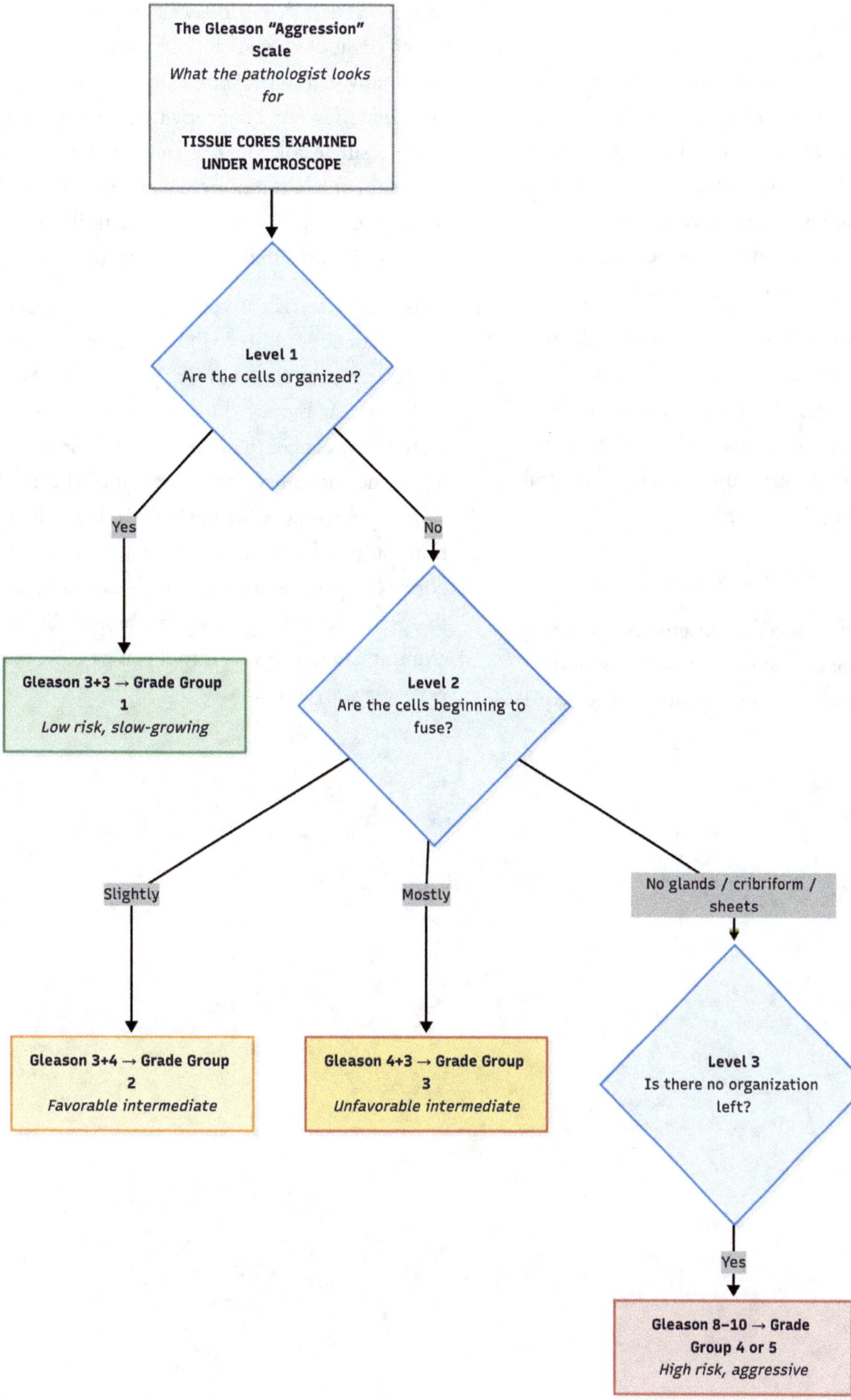
The Gleason "Aggression" Scale
What the pathologist looks for
TISSUE CORES EXAMINED UNDER MICROSCOPE
Level 1
Are the cells organized?
Yes
No
Gleason 3+3 → Grade Group 1
Low risk, slow-growing
Level 2
Are the cells beginning to fuse?
Slightly
Mostly
No glands / cribriform / sheets
Gleason 3+4 → Grade Group 2
Favorable intermediate
Gleason 4+3 → Grade Group 3
Unfavorable intermediate
Level 3
Is there no organization left?
Yes
Gleason 8–10 → Grade Group 4 or 5
High risk, aggressive

What Happens Next

Men with low grade, low volume prostate cancer are often good candidates for Active Surveillance. This approach involves regular PSA testing, periodic imaging, and occasional repeat biopsies. It allows men to avoid or delay aggressive treatments and their associated side effects while maintaining careful oversight.

When cancer is higher grade or more extensive, treatment is recommended more proactively. Options may include surgery, radiation therapy, medications, or combinations of these approaches. The biopsy findings play a central role in selecting the best plan.

Common Fears and Reassurances

Among all the cancers I diagnosed, prostate cancer is the one most often misunderstood by the patient receiving the diagnosis. The word cancer carries the same weight regardless of which organ it appears in, but the biology does not. Many of the prostate cancers I signed out are Grade Group 1, occupying a few millimeters in a single core out of twelve, with cells that look almost like the normal gland next door. A man with that diagnosis is statistically more likely to die with that cancer than from it.

This is why active surveillance exists as a serious, evidence-supported option, not a delay tactic. It means PSA checks, periodic imaging, and a repeat biopsy on a schedule. It means treating the cancer that needs treating and leaving alone the cancer that does not. The decision is yours and your urologist's, but the option only exists because someone took the cores, the pathologist read them carefully, and the grade came back low. The biopsy did not commit you to surgery. It told you whether surgery was warranted.

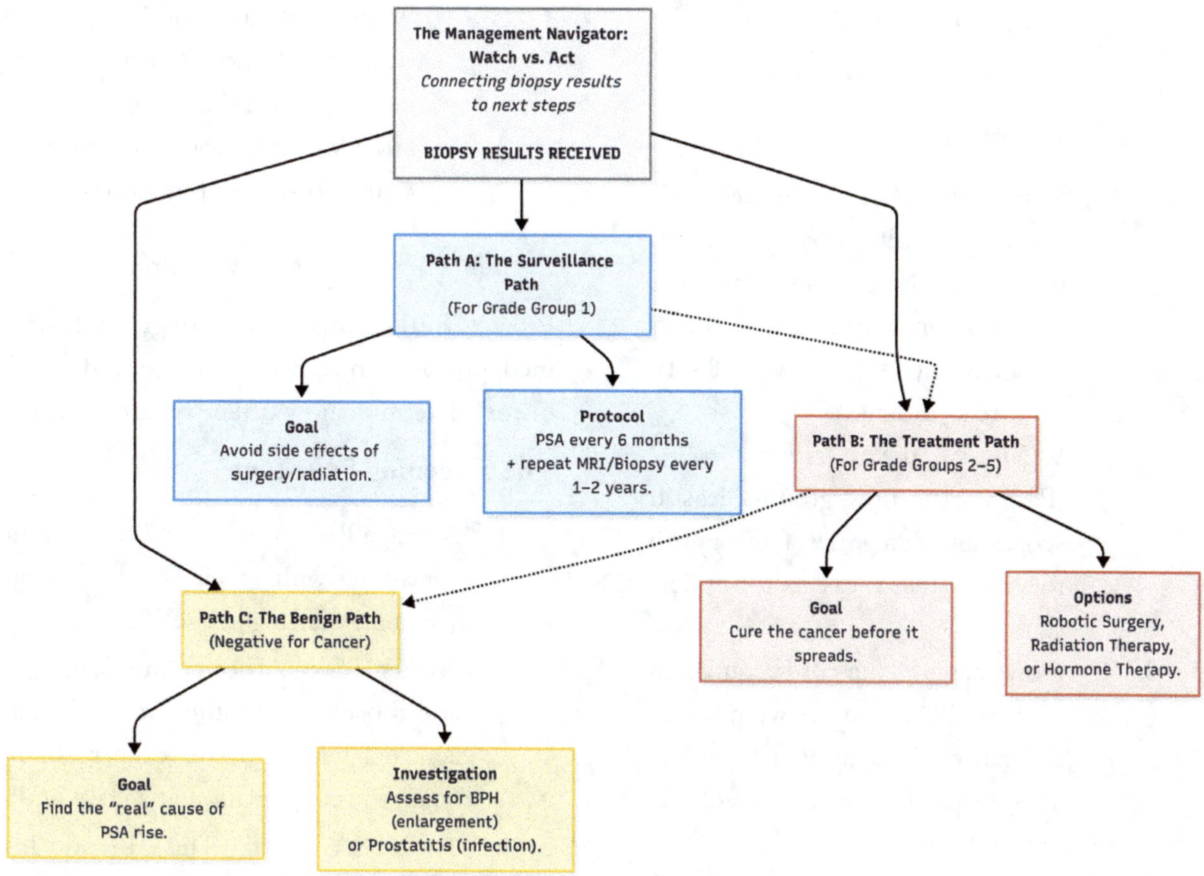

Example

Twelve biopsy cores were obtained, and three showed low grade cancer involving only small portions of the tissue. After reviewing the findings, the patient chose Active Surveillance. Several years later, there has been no progression and no treatment related side effects. His care was guided by the evidence the biopsy provided.

Author Tip: The 'Volume' Factor

Finding a small amount of Grade Group 1 in 1 out of 12 cores is very different than finding it in 10 out of 12 cores.

Pathologists call this 'tumor volume,' and it's a major factor in deciding if you can stay on Active Surveillance or if it's time to take action.

Questions to Ask Your Doctor During a Follow-up Appointment

Understanding the Pathology

1. What was the Gleason Score? (This is the most critical part of the report. It grades how aggressive the cells look on a scale of 6 to 10. A 6 is generally low-risk, while 8 - 10 is more aggressive.)
2. What is the Grade Group? (Pathologists now group Gleason scores into categories 1 through 5 to make them easier to understand.)
3. How many of the cores contained cancer? (If 12 samples were taken, did cancer show up in 1 or in 10? This helps determine the volume of the disease.)
4. Was there any Perineural Invasion? (This tells you if the cells are beginning to interact with the nerves surrounding the prostate.)

Determining the Cause

1. If it isn't cancer, what is causing my high PSA? (Is it BPH, an enlarged prostate, or Prostatitis, an infection/inflammation?)
2. Do these results suggest I need treatment right away, or am I a candidate for Active Surveillance?

Next Steps

1. Do I need further imaging, like a bone scan or a PSMA-PET scan, to see if the cells have moved elsewhere?
2. What are the pros and cons of my treatment options? (e.g., Surgery, radiation, or monitoring.)
3. How will this diagnosis affect my urinary or sexual function?

Recommended Prostate Exam Protocol

Prostate health is managed through a risk-stratified protocol, meaning your age and family history determine how often you are checked.

The Screening Start Line

- Average Risk: Men should have a conversation with their doctor about screening starting at age 50.
- Higher Risk: African American men and those with a father or brother diagnosed with prostate cancer should begin the conversation at age 40 or 45.
- The PSA Test: This blood test measures a protein made by the prostate. While not a cancer test, a rising number is a signal to investigate further.

The MRI-Fusion Protocol (MRI-Ultrasound Fusion Biopsy)

Modern protocol often involves a Prostate MRI before a biopsy.

- If the MRI shows a suspicious area (scored as a PI-RADS 4 or 5), the doctor uses fusion technology to overlay those images onto a live ultrasound during the biopsy.
- This ensures the needle targets the exact area of concern rather than sampling at random.

Management of Active Surveillance

If the biopsy shows a low-grade cancer (Gleason 6), the universal protocol is often Active Surveillance rather than immediate surgery. This involves:

- A PSA test every 6 months.
- A repeat biopsy or MRI every 1 to 2 years.
- This protocol aims to avoid the side effects of treatment while keeping a very close eye on the cells to ensure they don't become more aggressive.

Follow-up

If the biopsy is negative but the PSA remains high, the protocol dictates:

- Repeat PSA in 3 - 6 months.
- Biomarker tests (like 4Kscore or Prostate Health Index (PHI)) to see if a second biopsy is actually necessary.
- Continued Monitoring: A negative biopsy doesn't always mean the all clear if the PSA continues to climb; it may simply mean the needle missed a small area of concern.

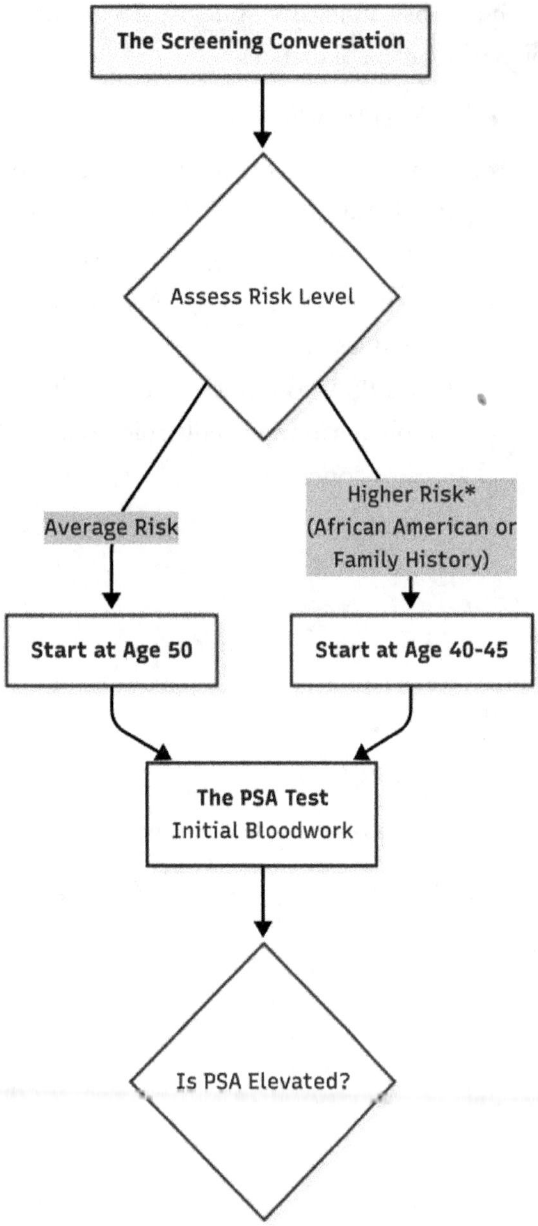
The Screening Conversation
Assess Risk Level
Average Risk
Higher Risk*
(African American or
Family History)
Start at Age 50
Start at Age 40-45
The PSA Test
Initial Bloodwork
Is PSA Elevated?

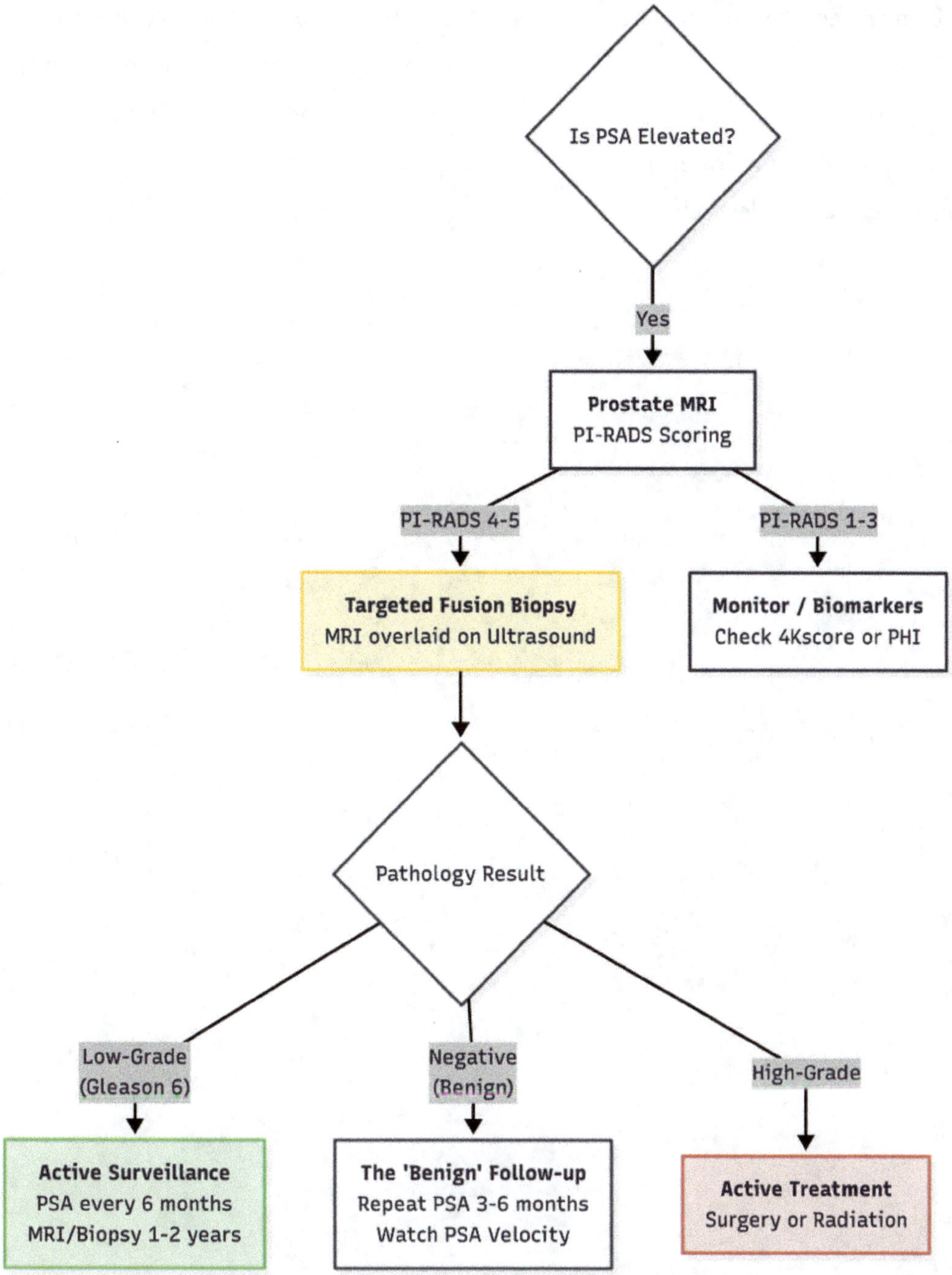

Quick Summary

- A prostate biopsy clarifies what a rising PSA or suspicious MRI actually means — PSA alone can rise from many non-cancer causes.
- The biopsy answers not just whether the diagnosis is cancer but how aggressive it is, using the Gleason / Grade Group system (1 = least aggressive, 5 = most).
- Many low-grade, low-volume cancers are best managed with Active Surveillance —

regular monitoring rather than immediate treatment.

- Transperineal and MRI-targeted approaches improve precision and lower infection risk compared with older techniques.
- Modern prostate care balances cancer control with quality of life; a cancer diagnosis does not automatically mean immediate surgery or radiation.

Chapter 13

Cervical Biopsies

Turning Screening Signals into Prevention

What It Is and Why It's Done

The cervix contains a biologically active region called the transformation zone. This is an area where one type of cell naturally changes into another over time. Because of this normal cell turnover, the transformation zone is particularly sensitive to infection with high-risk human papillomavirus, or HPV. In some people, persistent HPV infection can trigger abnormal cellular changes that develop gradually over years.

Cervical biopsies are most often performed after an abnormal Pap test, a positive high risk HPV test, or concerning findings during a pelvic exam. Importantly, many cervical abnormalities are temporary and resolve on their own without treatment. Others represent true precancerous changes that benefit from early intervention. A biopsy determines where a person falls along this spectrum, allowing care to be meticulously matched to the actual level of risk.

How the Biopsy Is Performed

Cervical biopsies are usually taken during a procedure called colposcopy. During colposcopy, the clinician uses a special microscope to closely examine the cervix. Gentle solutions are applied to the surface of the cervix that cause abnormal areas to stand out from healthy tissue.

Very small tissue samples are then taken from the areas that appear most suspicious. The procedure is brief. Some people feel mild cramping or a short pinching sensation during the biopsy, but discomfort is usually minimal and short lived. Most patients return to normal activities the same day.

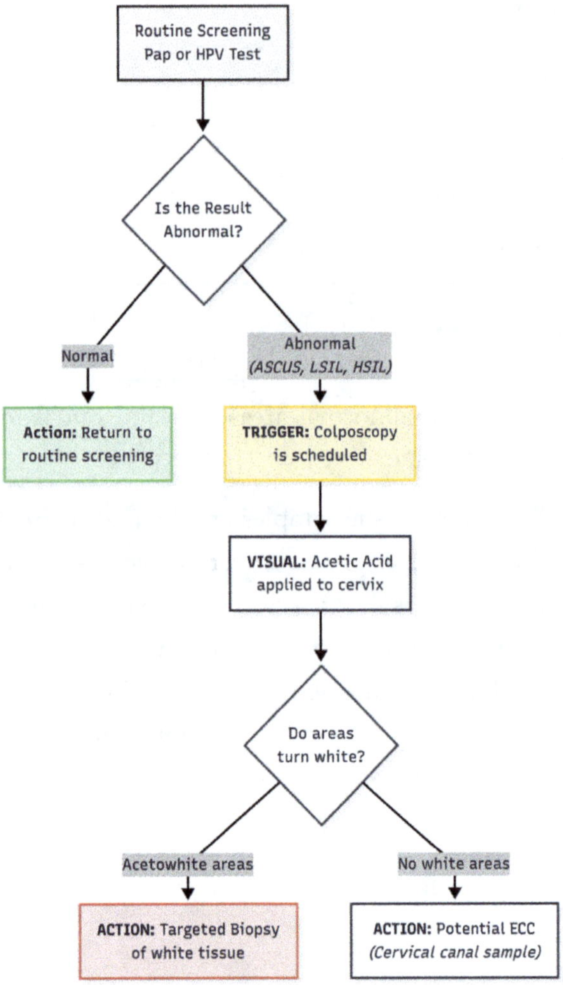

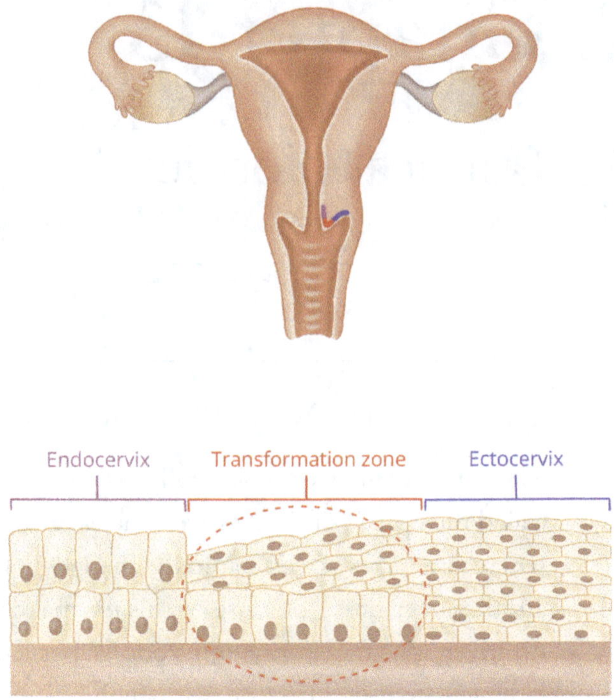

Figure 17. Cervical transformation zone illustrated

What the Pathologist Looks For

Under the microscope, cervical changes are graded according to severity. Mild changes, called low grade lesions, often reflect transient HPV effects and frequently resolve without treatment. Moderate and severe changes represent increasing levels of dysplasia, meaning abnormal cell development.

High grade dysplasia is considered true precancer. While it is not spreadable cancer, it has a meaningful risk of progressing if it is left untreated. The pathologist also carefully evaluates gland forming cells, which can develop a distinct type of precancer known as adenocarcinoma in situ. This condition requires particular attention and careful management.

If abnormal cells have crossed natural tissue boundaries and invaded deeper layers, the diagnosis is invasive cervical cancer. The purpose of biopsy is to identify changes well before this step occurs.

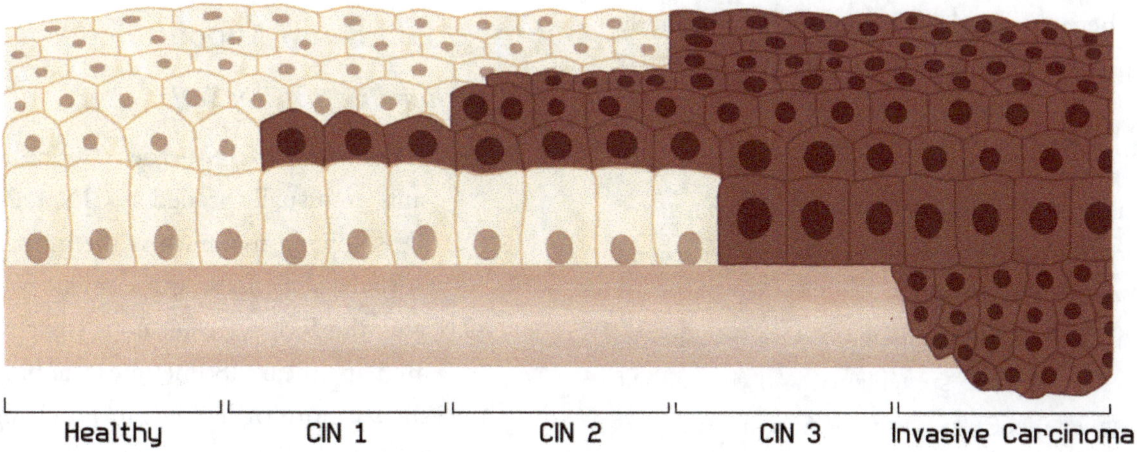

Figure 18. Illustration of cervical neoplasm from healthy to invasive cancer

How Results Are Reported

Cervical biopsy reports use standardized, widely accepted terminology so results can be interpreted consistently. Low grade findings often support observation rather than immediate treatment. High grade findings prompt treatment to prevent progression. Diagnoses involving glandular precancer or invasive cancer trigger definitive care planning.

When tissue has been removed, the report also indicates whether the abnormal area was completely excised by evaluating the edges of the specimen. This information helps determine whether additional treatment is necessary.

Each term in the report is meant to guide action.

What Happens Next

Low grade cervical changes are often managed with follow up testing and careful surveillance. High grade lesions are typically treated with localized procedures that remove abnormal tissue while preserving the structure and function of the cervix.

One common treatment is a loop excision procedure, which removes the affected area precisely and effectively. When invasive cancer is detected at an early stage, treatment begins promptly, and outcomes are often excellent.

Common Fears and Reassurances

Cervical screening is one of the quiet successes of modern medicine, and most patients do not realize they are inside that success when an abnormal result arrives. A generation ago, cervical cancer was a common and lethal disease. Today it is largely a disease we prevent. We do that by catching changes years, sometimes a decade, before they could become cancer.

When you receive an abnormal Pap result or a positive high-risk HPV test, it does not mean you have cancer. It means the system that was designed to find changes early found something worth a closer look. The biopsies that follow, taken during colposcopy, are typically tiny. Many show low-grade changes that the body will clear on its own. Some show high-grade dysplasia, which is treated with a localized procedure that removes the abnormal area and preserves the cervix. Either way, the process that began with the Pap test is doing exactly what it was built to do.

Example

A patient with persistent abnormal Pap test results underwent cervical biopsy, which showed high grade dysplasia. A cone biopsy removed the abnormal tissue with clear margins. She returned to routine surveillance and the risk of invasive cancer was stopped early, quietly, and effectively.

What This Means for You

Cervical biopsies are a cornerstone of modern cancer prevention. The Pap test detects an early signal; the colposcopic biopsy names what the signal means; a targeted procedure removes the abnormal tissue years before it could become invasive cancer. By the time you reach the biopsy, the system designed to protect you is already working.

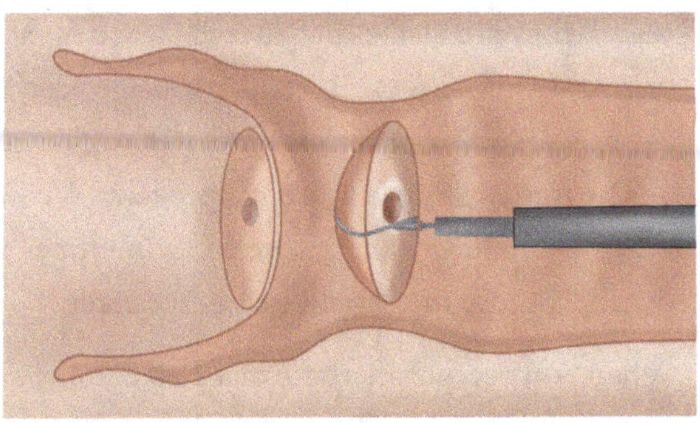

Figure 19. Cervical biopsy illustrated. See how a cone shaped cap of the cervix including transformation zone is removed with the LEEP tool.

Questions to Ask Your Doctor During a Follow-up Appointment

Understanding the CIN Scale

1. What was the CIN grade? (Cervical results are usually graded as CIN 1, 2, or 3. Knowing the grade is the most important factor in your treatment plan.)
2. Was the biopsy result consistent with my Pap smear? (Sometimes the biopsy shows more or less advanced changes than the initial screening.)
3. Were the margins clear? (If a larger piece was taken, like in a LEEP or Cone biopsy, you'll want to know if the abnormal area was completely removed.)

Linking to HPV

1. Did the biopsy show signs of high-risk types of HPV (Human Papillomavirus) infection?
2. Do I need a follow-up HPV test, or do we already know the strain?

Next Steps & Treatment

1. Do we watch and wait, or do we need to treat this now? (CIN 1 is often monitored, while CIN 2 or 3 usually requires a procedure.)
2. If treatment is needed, what are my options? (e.g., LEEP, cryotherapy, or laser therapy.)
3. How will this affect future pregnancies or my ability to carry a baby to term?
4. When is my next test of cure or follow-up Pap smear?

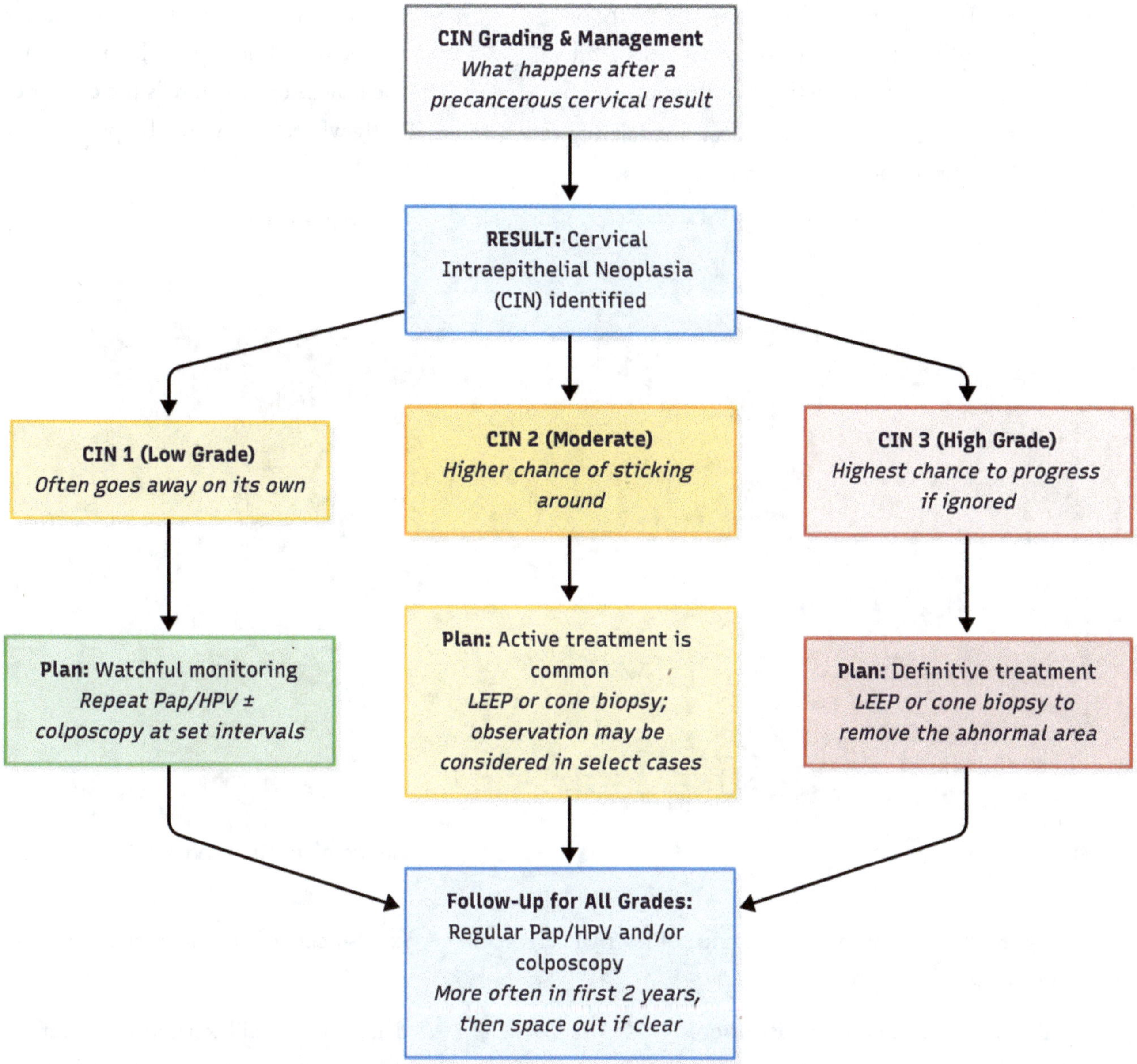

Recommended Cervical Exam Protocol

The protocol for cervical health is one of the most standardized in medicine, moving from general screening to targeted biopsy.

The Screening Schedule (The Primary Protocol)

- Age 21 - 29: Pap smear every 3 years. (HPV testing is usually only done if the Pap is abnormal).
- Age 30 - 65: The standard of care is co-testing (Pap + HPV test) every 5 years, or a Pap smear alone every 3 years.
- Over Age 65: Screening may stop if you have had regular normal results for the previous 10 years.

Colposcopy

- If a Pap smear shows ASCUS, LSIL, or HSIL (terms for abnormal cells), the protocol moves to a Colposcopy.
- The doctor uses a special magnifying lens to look at the cervix.
- They apply a vinegar-like solution (acetic acid); abnormal cells turn white (acetowhite), which tells the doctor exactly where to take the biopsy.

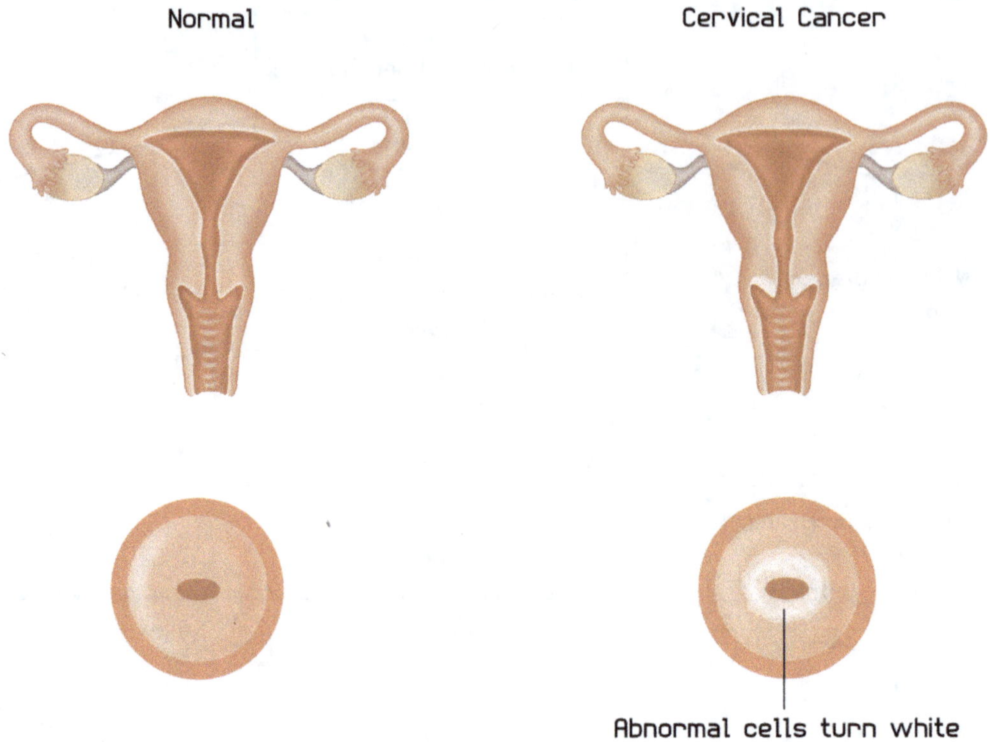

Figure 20. Colposcopy appearance of normal cervix and cervix with cancer after application of acetic acid.

The CIN Management Protocol

Once the biopsy results are in, doctors follow the ASCCP Guidelines:

- CIN 1 (Mild Dysplasia): Usually follows a monitor protocol. The body's immune system often clears these cells on its own. You will likely return in 6 - 12 months for a repeat Pap.
- CIN 2 or 3 (Moderate to Severe Dysplasia): These are considered precancerous. The protocol usually dictates removal of the tissue via LEEP (Loop Electrosurgical Excision Procedure) or a traditional Cone Biopsy surgically.

Post-Treatment Surveillance

After a procedure to remove abnormal cells, the protocol becomes more frequent. Patients treated for high-grade dysplasia require three (3) negative HPV-based tests or co-tests before they can return to extended screening intervals.

💡 **Author Tip: The 'Safety Line' (Basement Membrane)**

Think of the basement membrane as a floor. As long as abnormal cells are just standing on the floor (CIN 1–3),
they are precancerous and easily cleared away.

It only becomes 'invasive cancer' when those cells start digging through the floorboards into the rooms below.

Quick Summary

- A cervical biopsy follows an abnormal Pap test, a positive high-risk HPV test, or a concerning exam — it does not mean you have cancer.
- During colposcopy, a vinegar solution highlights abnormal areas so the most informative tissue can be sampled.
- Findings range from low-grade changes (CIN 1) that often resolve on their own to high-grade changes (CIN 2/3) that are treated to prevent cancer.
- Treatment (typically LEEP or cone biopsy) removes abnormal cells while preserving cervical structure and function.
- After treatment for high-grade disease, three negative HPV-based tests are required before returning to extended screening intervals.

Chapter 14

Thyroid Biopsies

Understanding Thyroid Nodules

What It Is and Why It's Done

Thyroid nodules are extremely common, especially as people get older. Many are discovered incidentally on imaging done for unrelated reasons, and most never cause symptoms or health problems. In fact, the vast majority of thyroid nodules are harmless.

A thyroid biopsy is performed to answer a focused and practical question: Is this nodule safe to monitor, or does it need treatment? Imaging can estimate risk based on size and appearance, but only a biopsy can examine the cells directly. The goal is not to rush into surgery, but to sort nodules that can be safely watched from those that deserve closer attention.

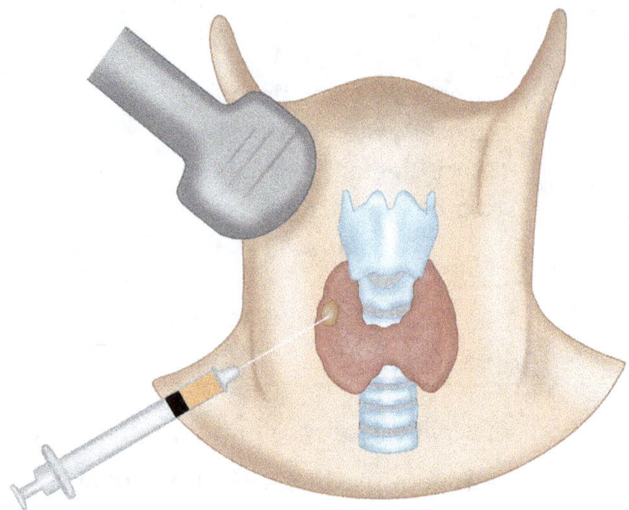

Figure 21. Ultrasound guided fine needle aspiration of thyroid

How the Biopsy Is Performed

Thyroid biopsies are typically done using ultrasound guidance, which allows precise placement of the needle into the nodule. A very thin needle is used to collect cells, fine needle aspiration (FNA).

Local numbing of the skin is usually sufficient. The needle is much thinner than those used for blood draws, and stitches are not required. The procedure is brief, and most people return to normal activities the same day with little more than mild soreness at the site.

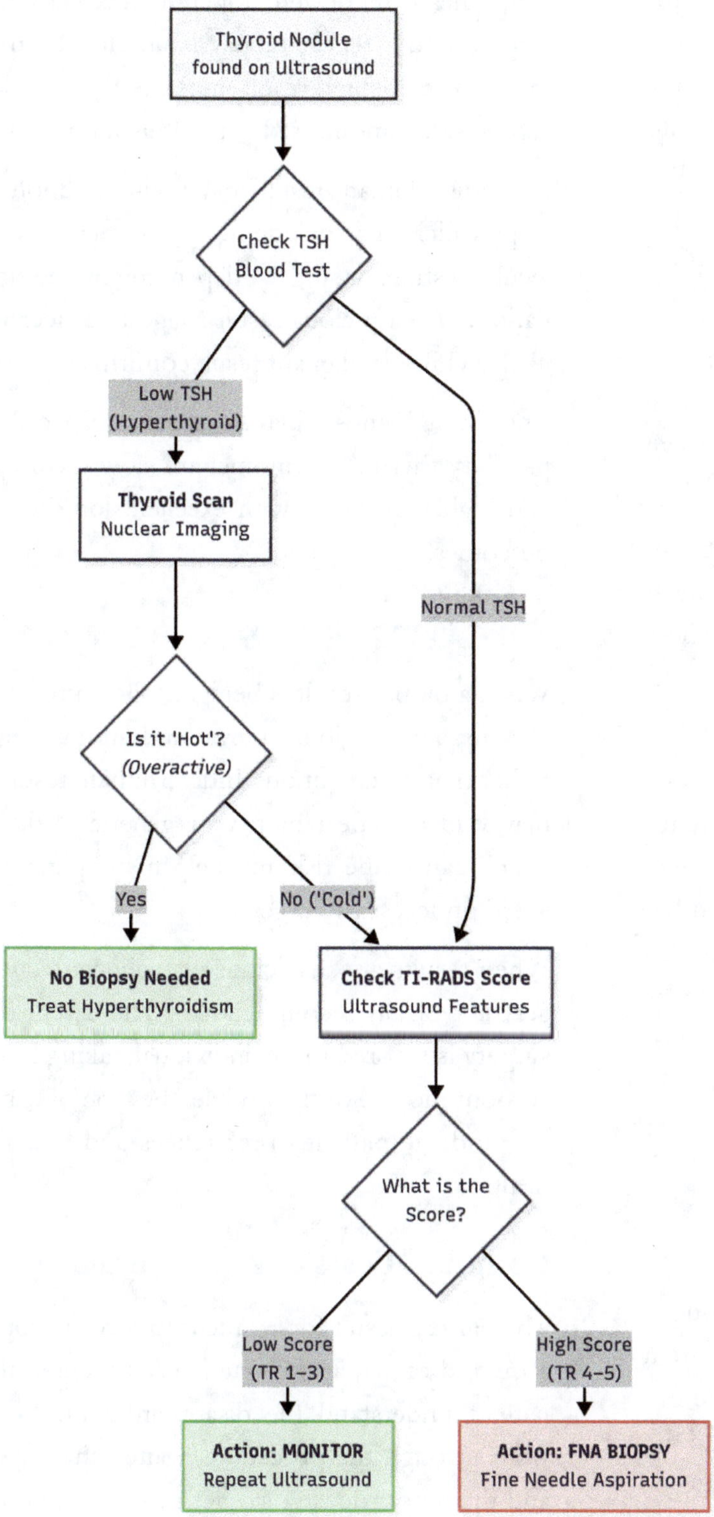

What the Pathologist Looks For

Because thyroid biopsies use FNA, the sample arrives as loose cells from the nodule rather than a coherent core, and that changes how the slides are prepared. The cells are spread onto glass slides so their details can be examined under the microscope. If enough material is available, extra cells may be saved for additional testing.

Some thyroid nodules show patterns that are clearly benign. These cells look orderly and mature, consistent with normal or overgrown thyroid tissue.

Other nodules display classic features of cancer, like a papillary thyroid carcinoma, the most common type of thyroid cancer. These changes are recognizable at the cellular level and allow a confident diagnosis.

Between these two ends of the spectrum lies a middle group of nodules that appear truly tumor like. These cells are neither clearly benign nor clearly malignant. The key distinction between benign and malignant tumors in this group depends on whether the growth invades its surrounding capsule or blood vessels. For this reason, some results are called indeterminate, reflecting a biological limitation rather than uncertainty or error.

How Results Are Reported

Thyroid biopsy results are reported using a standardized classification system. This system is designed to link what is seen under the microscope with the most likely outcome and the usual next steps. The system provides categories that guide decisions in a predictable way.

Thyroid biopsy results fall into a small number of well defined categories. A non diagnostic result means there were not enough cells to interpret, and a repeat biopsy is usually recommended. A benign result indicates the nodule can be safely monitored with ultrasound.

An indeterminate result may invite additional steps which may include repeat sampling, molecular testing, or surgery, depending on the situation. A suspicious result suggests cancer is likely, while a malignant result confirms cancer.

Importantly, most thyroid cancers, especially papillary thyroid carcinoma, are slow growing and highly treatable, with excellent long term outcomes.

What Happens Next

When a biopsy result is benign, follow up usually involves periodic ultrasound monitoring rather than intervention. Indeterminate results may lead to repeat biopsy or genetic testing, which can refine risk and help many patients avoid unnecessary surgery.

When results are suspicious or malignant, surgery is typically recommended. The extent of surgery is tailored to the individual, taking into account the size of the nodule, the type of cancer, and the patient's preferences and overall health.

Common Fears and Reassurances

The hardest result for a patient to receive from a thyroid biopsy is the one labeled indeterminate. I understand the disappointment. You went through the procedure, waited the days, and the report doesn't say yes or no. I want to explain what that result means from the microscope's side, because it is not a failure of the test.

A subset of thyroid nodules produce cells that, examined under any magnification, sit between the clearly benign and the clearly malignant. The only feature that would settle the question is whether those cells have broken through the capsule of the nodule, and that capsule is something I cannot see in an aspirate of loose cells. It would require the whole nodule on a slide. So when I write indeterminate, I am being honest about a limit of cellular evaluation, not guessing.

The good news is that we no longer have to send every indeterminate nodule to surgery. Molecular testing has become accurate enough to triage many of these toward observation, and many patients walk away with a benign genetic profile and an ultrasound schedule rather than a scar across their neck. The FNA, in other words, was not a wasted step. It was the test that got you a more targeted next test.

Example

A 1.7 centimeter thyroid nodule was biopsied and classified as indeterminate. Molecular testing showed a low risk genetic profile. Based on this information, the patient chose ultrasound monitoring rather than surgery and avoided an operation without compromising their health.

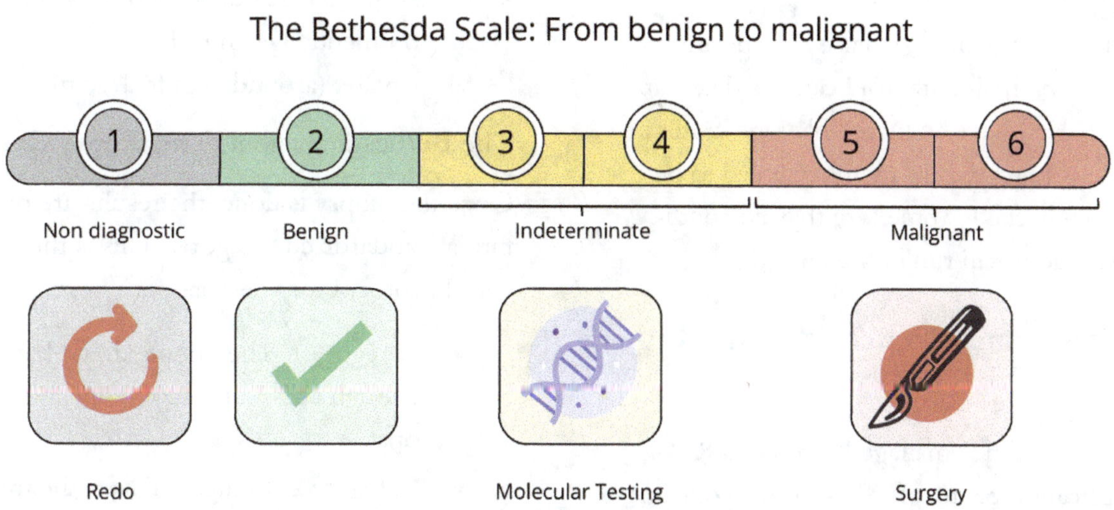

Figure 22. Illustration showing the Bethesda Scale and the subsequent next steps.

Questions to Ask Your Doctor During a Follow-up Appointment

Understanding the Results

1. What was the Bethesda Category of my result? This is the universal 1-through-6 grading system used for thyroid biopsies. Knowing your number is the most important piece of information you can have.
2. Is the nodule functioning or non-functioning? In other words, is this growth actually making thyroid hormone, or is it just a physical bump?

3. If the result was Indeterminate (Category 3 or 4), can we do molecular testing? Sometimes a biopsy doesn't give a yes or no answer. High-tech genetic tests can often look deeper into the sample to avoid an unnecessary surgery.

Next Steps and Management

1. Do I need surgery, or can we watch and wait? If the result is benign, ask if you can just monitor it with an ultrasound later on.
2. How often should I come back for a repeat scan? Is it in six months, a year, or longer?
3. Is the nodule large enough to affect my breathing or swallowing? Even if a nodule isn't cancer, its size can sometimes cause physical discomfort.

Long-Term Outlook

1. If it is cancer, what is the specific type? Most thyroid cancers (like Papillary) have an incredibly high cure rate.
2. Do my family members need to be checked? Some rare thyroid conditions can run in the family.

Recommended Thyroid Exam Protocol

Thyroid health is managed through a Risk-Stratification protocol. This means your doctor uses the physical features of the nodule to decide how often you need to be checked.

The Physical Neck Check

- The protocol usually starts with a simple exam where the doctor feels your neck while you swallow. If they feel a lump, or if you notice a fullness in your throat or a change in your voice, the next step is triggered.

The Ultrasound Protocol (TI-RADS)

Not every thyroid nodule needs a biopsy. Doctors use a system called TI-RADS to score a nodule based on how it looks on an ultrasound.

- TI-RADS 1 & 2: These look very safe. No biopsy is needed; just routine checks.
- TI-RADS 3: Low suspicion. A biopsy is usually only done if the nodule is quite large (over 2.5cm).
- TI-RADS 4 & 5: These have more suspicious features. A biopsy is recommended even if the nodule is smaller (around 1cm to 1.5cm).

The Bethesda System (The Biopsy Grade)

Once the biopsy is done, the results are put into a standardized category. This is the universal protocol for what happens next:

- Category 1: The sample didn't have enough cells. Protocol: Repeat the biopsy.
- Category 2 (Benign): This is the most common result. Protocol: Routine follow-up ultrasound in 12 to 24 months.
- Category 3 & 4 (Indeterminate): The cells look unusual but not definitely cancerous. Protocol: Genetic testing or removing half the thyroid to be safe.
- Category 5 & 6 (Malignant): This indicates cancer or a. high risk of it.

Protocol: Consultation with a surgeon for removal

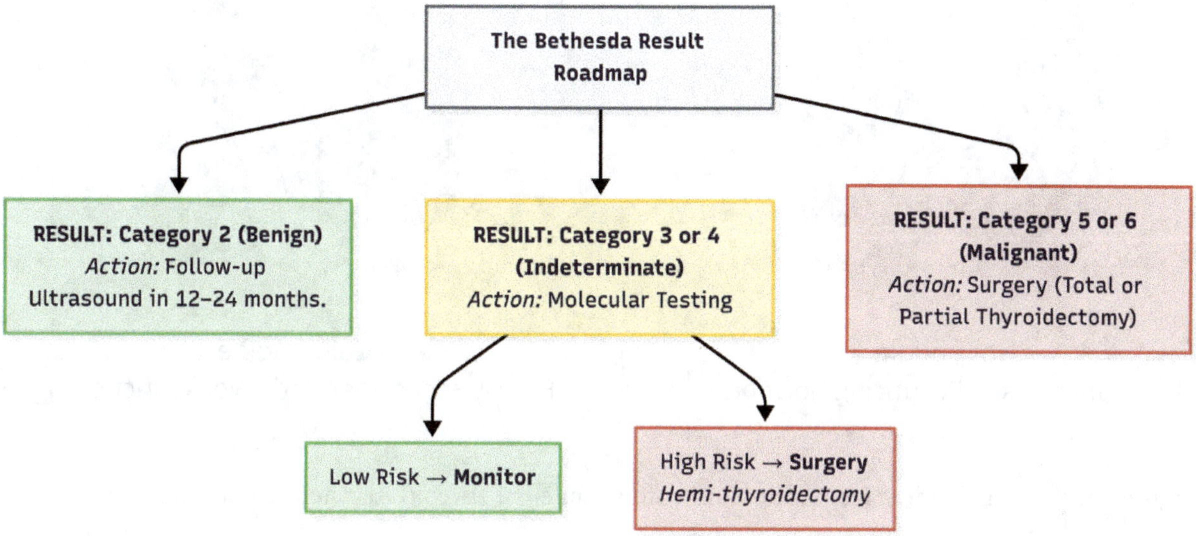

> **💡 Author Tip: The 'Sample Adequacy' Note**
>
> If your result is Category 1 (Non-diagnostic), don't worry – it doesn't mean anything is being hidden.
>
> It usually means the nodule was mostly fluid (a cyst) or there simply weren't enough cells to be certain.
>
> A repeat biopsy almost always solves the mystery.

The TSH Blood Test

A thyroid protocol is never complete without checking your hormone levels through a TSH (Thyroid Stimulating Hormone) test.

- If your TSH is low (Hyperthyroidism), your nodule might be hot, meaning it's overactive. Interestingly, hot nodules are almost never cancerous and often don't even need a needle biopsy!
- If your TSH is normal, the doctor relies strictly on the ultrasound and biopsy findings.

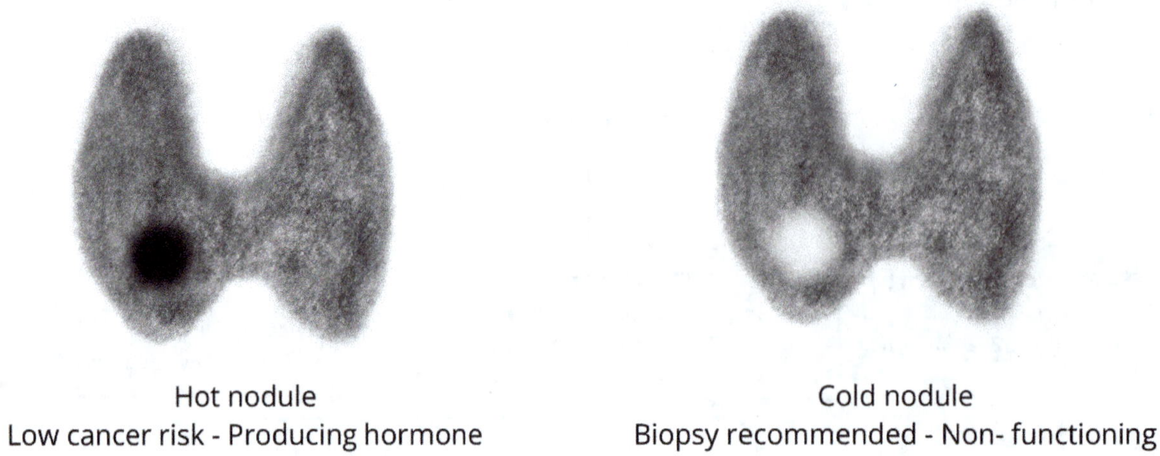

Figure 23. Imaging appearance of hot and cold nodules of thyroid that help determine whether a biopsy is recommended or not.

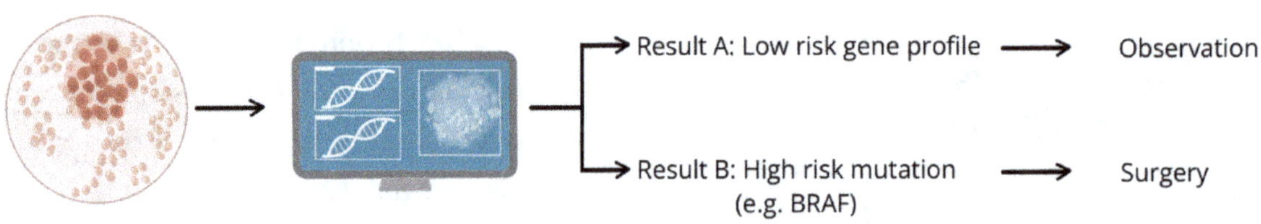

Figure 24. Illustration showing how gene profile result helps next step determination

Quick Summary

- Most thyroid nodules are harmless; an FNA biopsy answers whether yours is safe to monitor or needs treatment, not whether you have cancer.
- The procedure uses a needle thinner than a standard blood draw, takes only minutes, and does not require stitches.
- Results are reported using the Bethesda system (categories 1–6) which directly maps to the next step, from monitoring to surgery.
- About one in four biopsies returns "indeterminate" — this reflects biology, not error. Molecular testing can often resolve it without surgery.
- Most thyroid cancers (especially papillary) are slow-growing with excellent long-term outcomes when treated.

Chapter 15

Oral Cavity Biopsies

Lips, Tongue, Cheeks, and the Floor of the Mouth

What It Is and Why It's Done

The mouth is one of the most active and exposed parts of the body. Every day it encounters heat from food and drinks, constant friction from chewing and speaking, and a wide range of substances, from spices and alcohol to tobacco and dental products. Because of this continual exposure, changes in the lining of the mouth are common.

White patches, red areas, sores that do not heal, or small lumps can look very similar on the surface even though their causes may be very different (figure 25). Some changes are due to irritation, infection, or inflammation. Others represent precancerous changes, and a small number are early cancers.

A biopsy is the only reliable way to tell the difference. A biopsy allows reassuring findings to be confirmed and concerning changes to be addressed early, when treatment is simplest and outcomes are best.

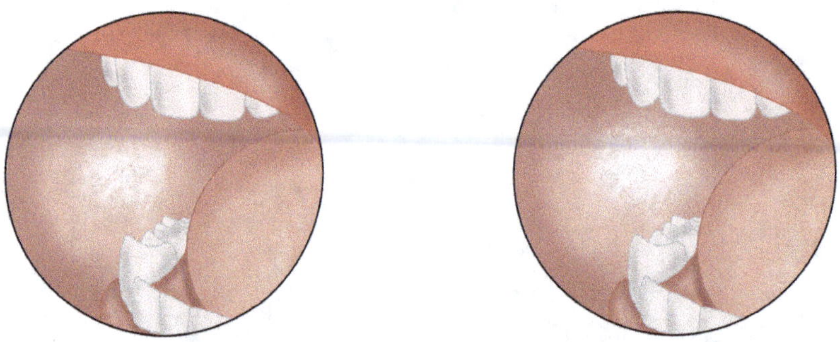

Frictional Keratosis (Benign)
Thickened white surface caused by jagged tooth rubbing the teeth

Leukoplakia (Precancerous)
Similar white patch caused by cell mutation

Figure 25. Oral lesions may look the same to the naked eye. But microscopic appearance of the biopsy will tell them apart.

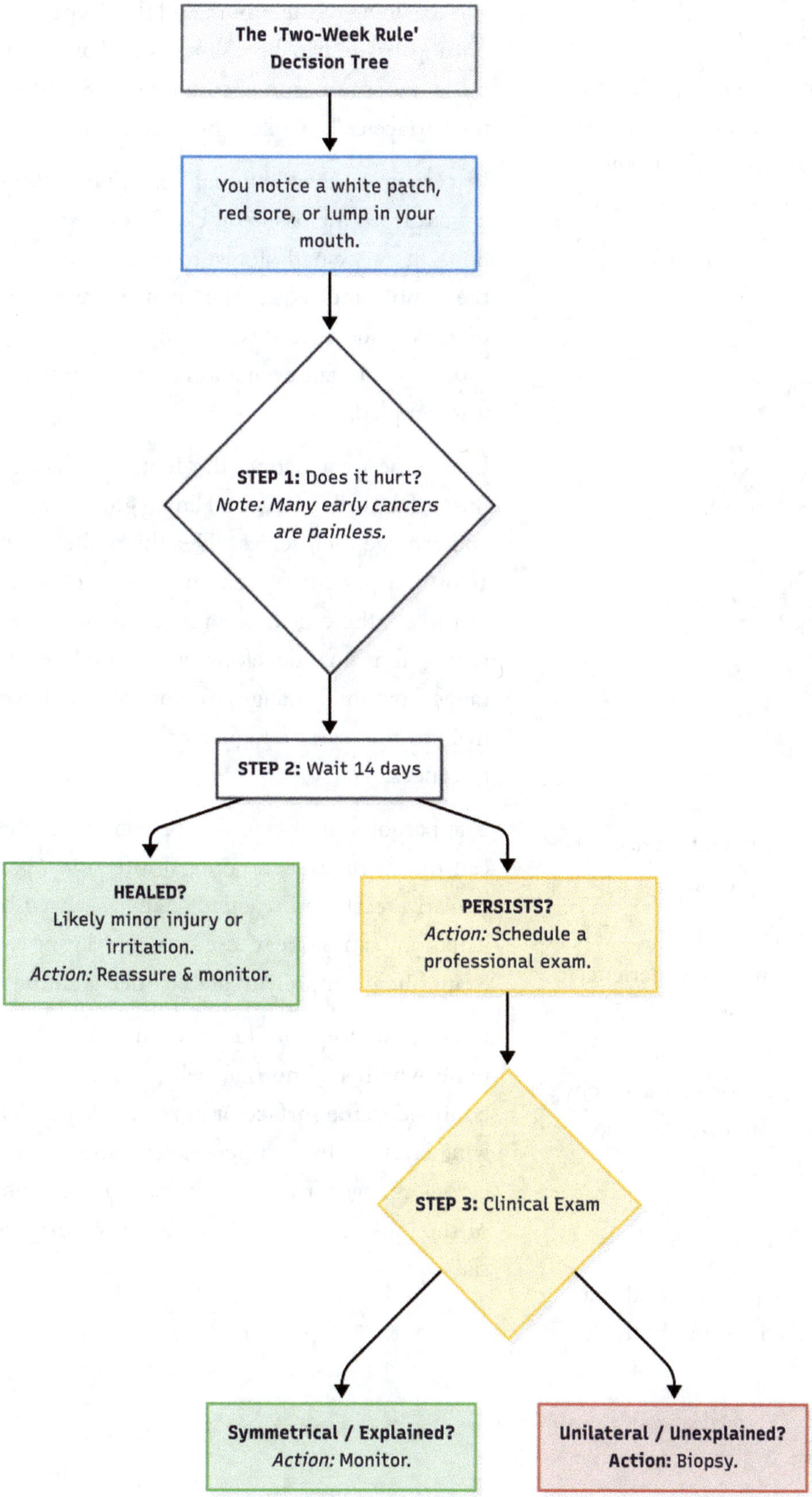
The 'Two-Week Rule' Decision Tree
You notice a white patch, red sore, or lump in your mouth.
STEP 1: Does it hurt? Note: Many early cancers are painless.
STEP 2: Wait 14 days
HEALED? Likely minor injury or irritation. Action: Reassure & monitor.
PERSISTS? Action: Schedule a professional exam.
STEP 3: Clinical Exam
Symmetrical / Explained? Action: Monitor.
Unilateral / Unexplained? Action: Biopsy.

How the Biopsy Is Performed

Oral cavity biopsies are usually quick and straightforward. The area of concern is first numbed with a local anesthetic, which keeps discomfort to a minimum. A small piece of tissue, often only a few millimeters in size, is then removed.

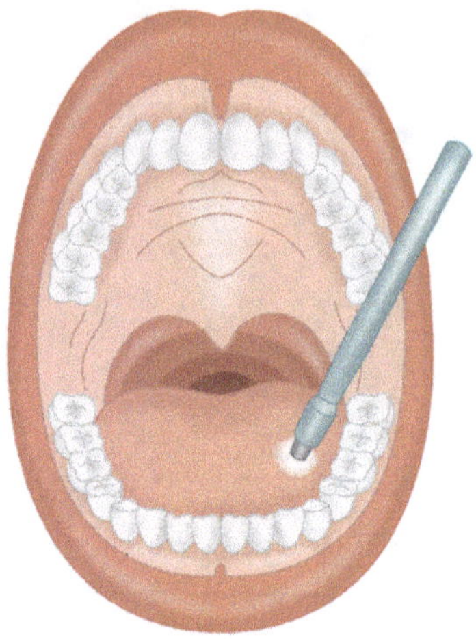

Figure 26. Punch biopsy of a white lesion of the tongue using punch biopsy tool.

The procedure itself typically takes only a few minutes. Afterwards, most people experience mild soreness, similar to a minor mouth ulcer. Healing usually occurs over several days. In some locations or for larger biopsies, a stitch may be placed, but stitches are often not necessary.

What the Pathologist Looks For

Once the biopsy reaches the pathology laboratory, it is carefully processed so that both the surface lining of the mouth and the deeper supporting tissue can be examined. This is important because some conditions affect only the surface cells, while others extend deeper.

In certain cases, additional very thin sections are cut from the tissue block. These extra sections allow the pathologist to examine more of the sample and reduce the chance that a small or focal abnormality is missed. The goal is a thorough and fair evaluation of everything that was sampled.

Under the microscope, the first focus is how the surface cells of the oral lining grow, mature, and arrange themselves. Healthy tissue shows an orderly pattern. When this process becomes disrupted, the cells may show dysplasia, which means abnormal development. Dysplasia can range from mild changes to more severe abnormalities that carry a higher risk of progressing to cancer.

The pathologist also looks for conditions that can mimic precancer. Fungal infections, particularly yeast, and reactive changes caused by irritation can appear concerning during an exam but are entirely treatable once identified.

Finally, the deeper tissue is evaluated to determine whether abnormal cells, if any, remain confined to the surface or have invaded underlying layers. This distinction separates precancerous changes from invasive cancer and is one of the most important features of the diagnosis.

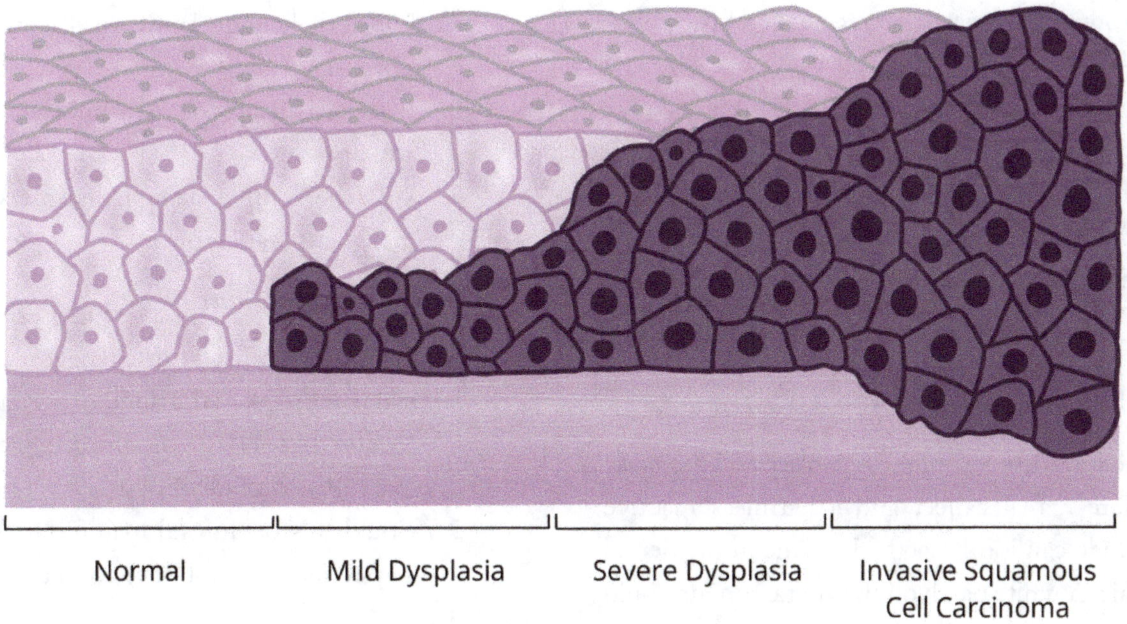

Figure 27. Illustration of microscopic changes seen from normal lining to a cancerous lining.

How Results Are Reported

In the pathology reports pertinent findings (neoplasm, irritation or infection) are clearly identified and named. Dysplasia is graded as mild, moderate, or high grade, reflecting how abnormal the cells appear and how likely they are to progress if left untreated.

High grade dysplasia is treated proactively because removing it prevents progression to cancer. If abnormal cells have broken through normal tissue boundaries and invaded deeper layers, the diagnosis is invasive squamous cell carcinoma, the most common cancer of the oral cavity. This diagnosis leads to timely treatment planning and coordinated care.

What Happens Next

When the biopsy shows irritation or infection, treatment usually involves local care, such as medication or removal of the source of irritation. Precancerous lesions, particularly those with higher grade dysplasia, are typically removed to eliminate future risk.

When oral cancer is detected early, treatment can begin promptly. Early diagnosis often allows for simpler procedures, better preservation of speech and swallowing, and excellent outcomes. The earlier a true problem is identified, the more options are available and the better the results tend to be.

Example

A rough white patch on the inside of the cheek raised concern for cancer. Biopsy showed moderate dysplasia, a precancerous change without invasion. The area was remove which effectively avoided progression. What initially looked ambiguous became a manageable and preventable problem once the correct diagnosis was made.

What This Means for You

The mouth is one of the few places on the body where a real cancer and a harmless reactive change can look exactly the same in the dental chair. A white patch on the lateral tongue could be from chronic biting against an uneven molar, or it could be a high-grade dysplasia three years away from squamous cell carcinoma. On the slide, the two are unmistakable. Without the slide, they are a coin flip.

That is the practical case for a small biopsy of any oral lesion that has not healed after about two weeks. The procedure is brief: a few minutes in a dental or ENT chair, a numb spot afterward that feels like a self-inflicted bite for a day or two. The information it returns can be decisive. The earliest oral cancers, caught while still confined to the surface lining, are often treated with a single localized procedure and excellent long-term outcomes. The same disease two years later, having reached the muscle of the tongue or the floor of the mouth, is a different conversation entirely.

Questions to Ask Your Doctor During a Follow-up Appointment

Clarifying the Results

1. What is the specific name of the lesion or condition found? (e.g., Is it leukoplakia, lichen planus, or a common fibroma?)
2. If there is dysplasia: is it mild, moderate, or severe?
3. Was the sample benign (harmless) or malignant (cancerous)?

Understanding the Cause

1. What likely caused this change? (e.g., Is it related to dental irritation, a viral infection like HPV, or lifestyle factors like tobacco or alcohol use?)
2. Could this be an oral manifestation of a systemic (whole-body) condition?

Next Steps & Management

1. Does the entire lesion need to be removed, or is monitoring enough?
2. What is the risk of this coming back or progressing?
3. Do I need to see a specialist, such as an Oral Surgeon or an Ear, Nose, and Throat (ENT) doctor?
4. How should I care for the site while it heals? (Ask about specific mouthwashes or foods to avoid.)

Recommended Oral Exam Protocol

Dentists and oral surgeons follow a standardized protocol to ensure that oral cancers, which are often painless in early stages, are caught early.

The Regular Dental Screening (Every 6 Months)

- The most common protocol is the professional oral cancer screening performed during your biannual dental cleaning.

- The Feel and Look Method: The provider should palpate (feel) your jaw and neck for lumps and visually inspect the tongue (pulling it forward with gauze), the roof and floor of the mouth.

The Monthly Self-Exam

Once a month, use a bright light and a mirror to look for:

- Texture Changes: Look for lumps, thickened skin, or crusty areas that feel different from the surrounding tissue.
- The Two-Week Rule: Any sore, red patch, or white patch that does not heal within 14 days should be professionally evaluated.

High-Risk Surveillance

If you have a history of heavy tobacco use, significant alcohol consumption, or a previous diagnosis of oral dysplasia, the protocol shifts:

- Frequent Checks: Exams may be required every 3 to 6 months.
- Advanced Tools: Some clinicians use specialized lights (like VELscope) or brush biopsies to identify abnormal metabolic activity in the tissue before it is visible to the naked eye.

The Symmetry Check

The oral cavity is generally symmetrical, so something that appears only on one side, like a patch, lump, or sore, often deserves closer attention. While not an official rule, clinicians commonly treat unilateral lesions as potentially significant and may recommend a prompt evaluation or biopsy, depending on how it looks and whether it persists.

> 💡 **Author Tip: The 'Symmetry' Check**
>
> Think symmetrically: The body generally likes to be even.
>
> If you have a bump on both sides of your tongue in the same spot, it's likely normal anatomy.
>
> If you have a sore on only one side – without a 'twin' on the other – that is the one your dentist will examine most closely.

Quick Summary

- The mouth lining is exposed to constant friction, heat, and chemicals. Persistent white patches, red areas, or sores that don't heal in two weeks need professional evaluation.
- A biopsy is the only reliable way to distinguish irritation, infection, precancer, and early cancer — they can look identical to the eye.
- The pathologist grades any dysplasia (abnormal development) as mild, moderate, or high-grade. High-grade dysplasia is treated proactively to prevent cancer.

- Early oral cancers caught at the precancerous stage are typically treated with simple procedures that preserve speech and swallowing.
- Twice-yearly dental visits include oral cancer screening; high-risk patients (tobacco, alcohol, prior dysplasia) may need exams every 3–6 months.

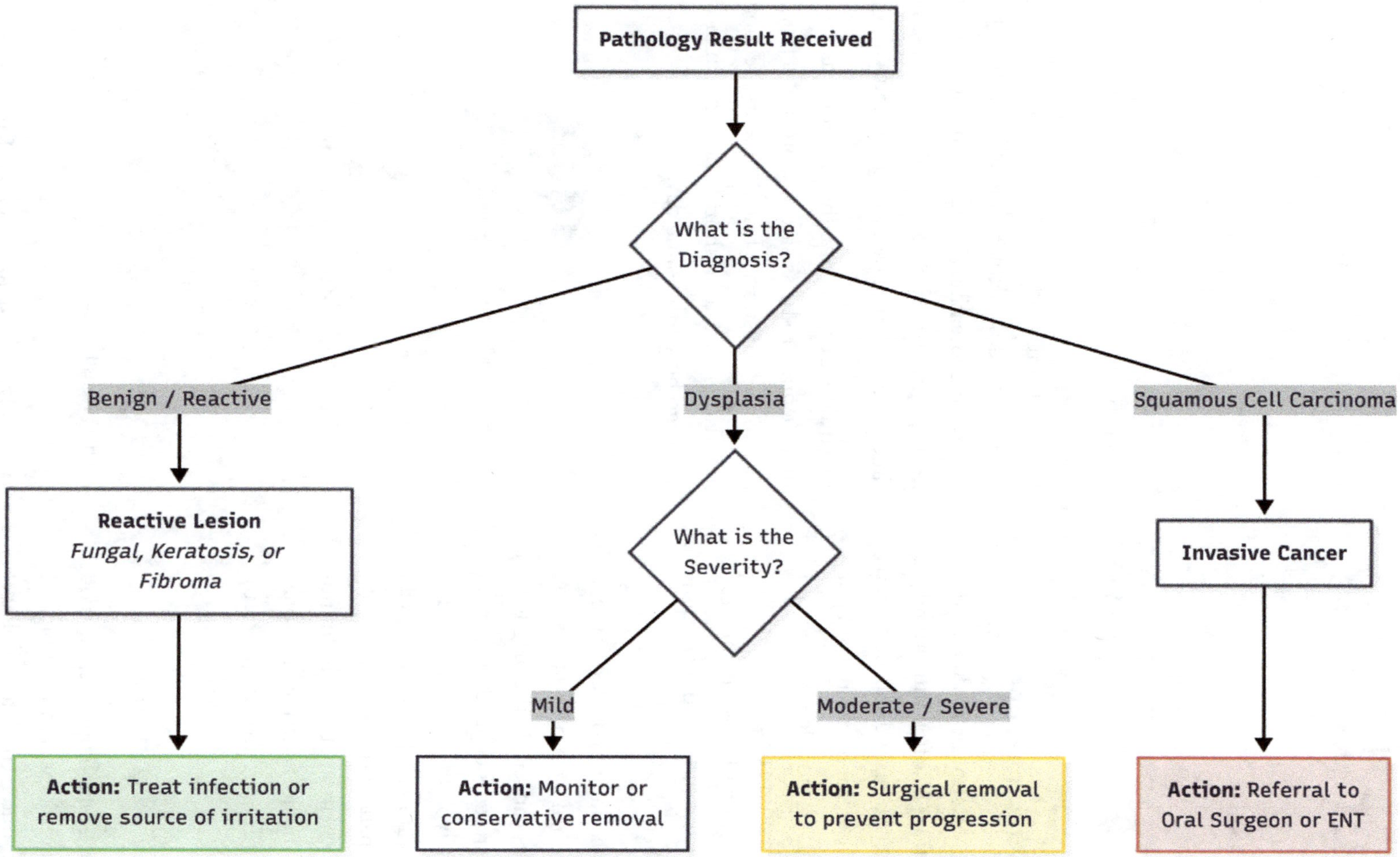
Pathology Result Received
What is the Diagnosis?
Benign / Reactive
Dysplasia
Squamous Cell Carcinoma
Reactive Lesion
Fungal, Keratosis, or Fibroma
What is the Severity?
Invasive Cancer
Mild
Moderate / Severe
Action: Treat infection or remove source of irritation
Action: Monitor or conservative removal
Action: Surgical removal to prevent progression
Action: Referral to Oral Surgeon or ENT

Chapter 16

Lung Biopsy

Small Samples, Big Answers

What It Is and Why It's Done

When imaging reveals a spot or nodule in the lung, the first reaction is often uncertainty. Scans can show size, shape, and location, but they cannot reliably determine what the spot represents. Many lung nodules are benign scars, areas of inflammation, or infection. Others may be cancer. A lung biopsy is the step that provides certainty by allowing direct examination of the cells themselves.

In modern medicine, lung biopsies serve a broader purpose than simply answering whether the finding is cancer. If the diagnosis is cancer, today's treatments depend heavily on identifying the exact type of lung cancer and, often, its molecular features. These details can determine whether a patient is best treated with surgery, radiation, chemotherapy, immunotherapy, or targeted medications taken as pills. Even very small samples can provide powerful guidance.

How the Biopsy Is Performed

The method used for a lung biopsy depends on where the abnormality sits within the lung. If the spot is near the outer edge, a radiologist may guide a thin needle through the chest wall using CT imaging. When the area is deeper or closer to the airways, a pulmonologist may reach it from inside the lung using bronchoscopy (a flexible camera passed through the mouth and breathing tubes). In some cases, nearby lymph nodes are sampled at the same time to see whether disease has spread.

Regardless of the route, the procedure is carefully planned to be as safe and precise as possible. Most biopsies are brief. Patients are monitored afterward for a short period and, in most cases, go home the same day.

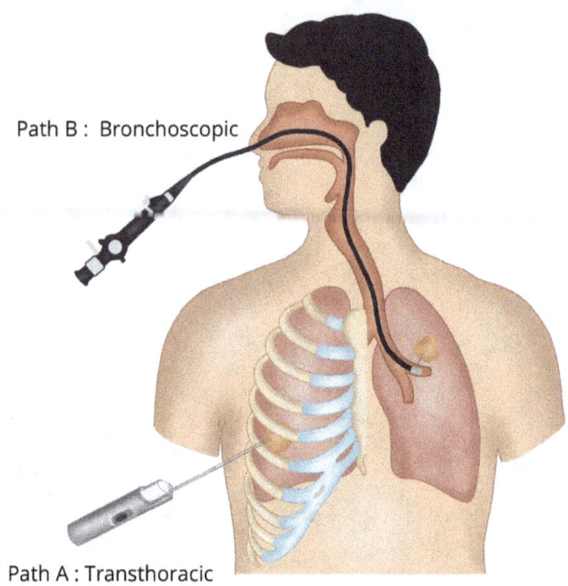

Figure 28. Bronchoscopic and transthoracic lung biopsy illustrations.

What the Pathologist Looks For

Part of the planning behind a lung biopsy is ensuring that enough material is collected to run the tests that matter most. This often allows diagnosis, special stains, and genetic testing to be completed without the need for repeat procedures.

The first question the pathologist answers is whether the finding is benign or malignant. When the diagnosis is cancer, the next step is determining whether it started in the lung or spread there from another organ.

For cancers that originate in the lung, the pathologist identifies the specific type, most commonly adenocarcinoma or squamous cell carcinoma. These distinctions matter because treatments differ. Once the type is established, additional tests may be performed to look for markers or genetic changes that predict which therapies are most likely to work best. The report names what was found in direct terms, along with the supporting molecular results.

What Happens Next

Your medical team combines the biopsy results with imaging studies and your overall health to choose the most appropriate next step. For some patients, surgery or focused radiation may be the best option. For others, targeted medicines or immunotherapy offer effective control with fewer side effects. In many cases, a combination of approaches is used.

The biopsy ensures that treatment is chosen thoughtfully, based on the biology of the tumor.

Common Fears and Reassurances

Two fears come up before nearly every lung biopsy: the fear that the needle will hurt, and the fear that despite everything, the sample will not be enough. Both are worth taking seriously, and both have changed in the last decade in ways worth knowing.

For pain, the needle path is numbed thoroughly, and many patients receive light sedation as well. The sharp sensation people describe is usually the initial anesthetic, not the biopsy itself. A small pneumothorax — air leaking into the chest cavity — happens in a minority of cases and almost always resolves on its own with observation. The post-procedure chest X-ray is a check, not an alarm.

For sample adequacy, the modern tools have closed most of the gap. CT guidance and navigational bronchoscopy let the radiologist or pulmonologist watch the needle approach the nodule in real time. When I receive the cores, I am often comparing what is on the slide against the radiologist's image side by side, and I will say so in the report if I do not think the tissue captured the lesion. If we did not get enough, we say so plainly and try again. That honesty is built into the workflow precisely because the stakes of the next conversation are high.

Example

A small lung nodule was biopsied and found to be adenocarcinoma with a specific genetic change. Instead of chemotherapy, the patient started a targeted pill designed for that alteration. The tumor shrank quickly, and treatment was well tolerated.

What This Means for You

A lung biopsy transforms an unclear image into a clear plan. It answers whether a finding is cancer, identifies what kind, and reveals which treatments are most likely to help. A tiny sample can make a decisive difference.

Questions to Ask Your Doctor During a Follow-up Appointment

Clarifying the Results

1. What is the specific name of the finding? (e.g., Is it a granuloma from an old infection, or a specific type of cancer like adenocarcinoma?)
2. If it is an infection, exactly what organism is causing it? (This ensures you get the right antibiotic or antifungal.)
3. Was the sample adequate? (Lung samples can be small; ask if there was enough tissue to run all the necessary tests.)

Next Steps & Management

1. What is the Stage and Grade? (Stage tells you if it has spread; Grade tells you how fast the cells are likely to grow.)
2. Have Biomarker tests been performed? (These are high-tech tests that look for genetic switches in the cells that can be turned off with targeted pills rather than traditional chemotherapy.)
3. Do I need a PET scan or a brain MRI?

Recommended Lung Exam Protocol

The protocol for lung health is centered on early detection in those with a history of smoking, as well as a strict system for tracking accidental findings in non-smokers.

The High-Risk Screening (LDCT)

The universal gold standard for lung cancer prevention is the Annual Low-Dose CT (LDCT) scan. This is recommended for individuals who meet the Triple-A criteria:

- Age: 50 to 80 years old.
- Amount: A 20 pack-year smoking history (e.g., 1 pack a day for 20 years).
- Active/Recent: Currently smoke or have quit within the last 15 years.

The Nodule Watchlist (Lung-RADS)

If a scan shows a spot, doctors follow the Lung-RADS protocol to decide how often to check it. This prevents unnecessary biopsies while ensuring dangerous spots don't get ignored:

- Category 1 & 2 (Small/Stable): Continue annual screening.
- Category 3 (Intermediate): Repeat the scan in 6 months to check for any growth.
- Category 4 (Suspicious): Proceed to a biopsy or a PET scan immediately.

The Two-Year Rule

In the world of lung pathology, a nodule that remains the exact same size for two years on CT scans is almost universally considered benign (non-cancerous). If your spot hasn't changed in two years, your care team may move from active concern to routine monitoring.

Post-Procedure Safety

Because the lungs are like delicate balloons, the protocol after a needle biopsy includes a safety check:

- Observation: You will stay for a few hours to ensure your breathing is stable.
- X-ray Check: A quick chest X-ray is often taken to ensure no air leaked out of the lung (a condition called a pneumothorax) during the sampling.

> 💡 **Author Tip: The 'Adequacy' Balance**
>
> **Small Sample, Big Job:** Lung biopsies are often tiny, sometimes the size of a grain of rice.
>
> Because so many molecular tests are required today, the pathologist's biggest challenge is *'tissue stewardship.'*
>
> If your report says **'Insufficient for molecular testing'**, it simply means the tissue ran out before all DNA studies could be completed.
>
> A repeat biopsy may be needed to get the full roadmap.

Quick Summary

- A lung biopsy turns an unclear nodule on a scan into a clear diagnosis. Many nodules are scars or infections; some are cancer.
- The route depends on location — through the chest wall under CT guidance for outer nodules, through the airways via bronchoscopy for deeper ones.
- Modern lung biopsies provide tissue not only for diagnosis but for molecular testing that determines whether targeted pills or immunotherapy will work better than chemotherapy.
- The most common complication is a small lung air leak (pneumothorax), usually minor and self-resolving, with a chest X-ray taken afterward as a safety check.
- A nodule unchanged in size for two years on CT is almost always benign.

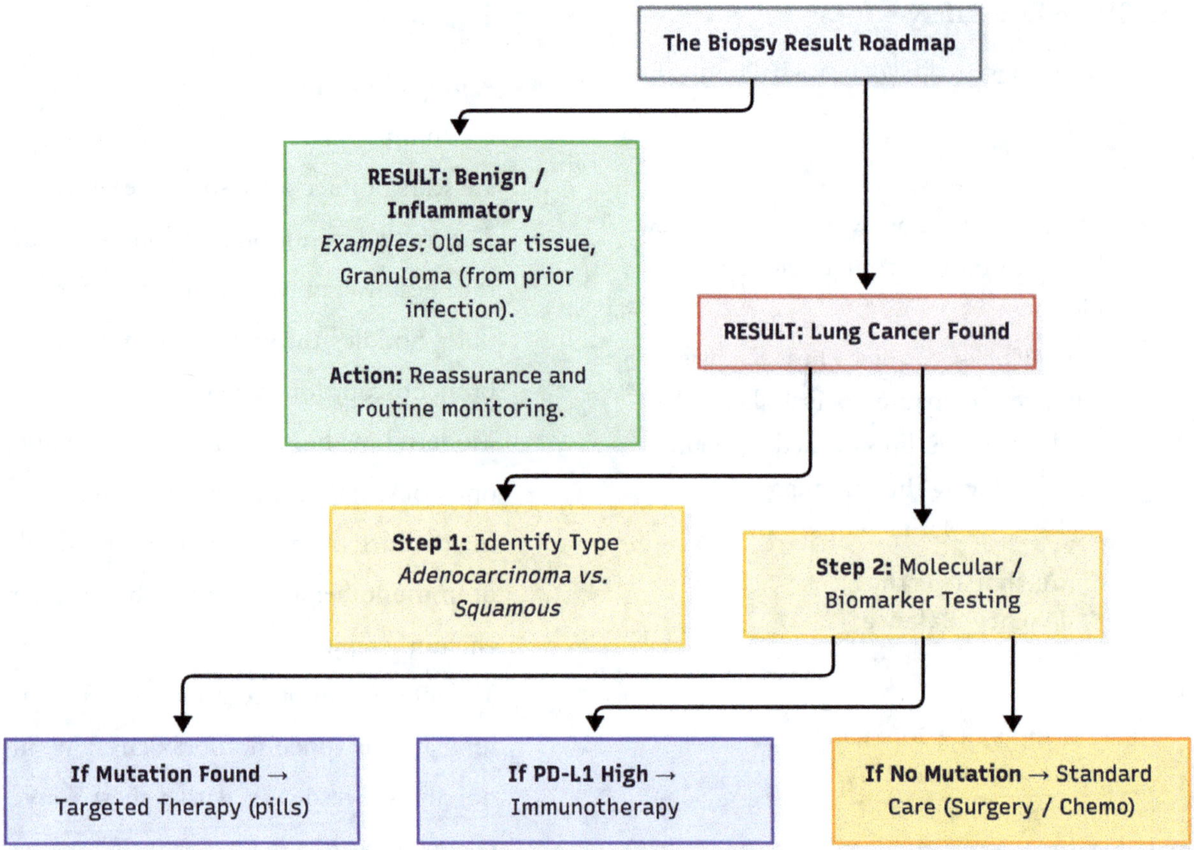
The Biopsy Result Roadmap
RESULT: Benign / Inflammatory
Examples: Old scar tissue, Granuloma (from prior infection).
Action: Reassurance and routine monitoring.
RESULT: Lung Cancer Found
Step 1: Identify Type
Adenocarcinoma vs. Squamous
Step 2: Molecular / Biomarker Testing
If Mutation Found → Targeted Therapy (pills)
If PD-L1 High → Immunotherapy
If No Mutation → Standard Care (Surgery / Chemo)

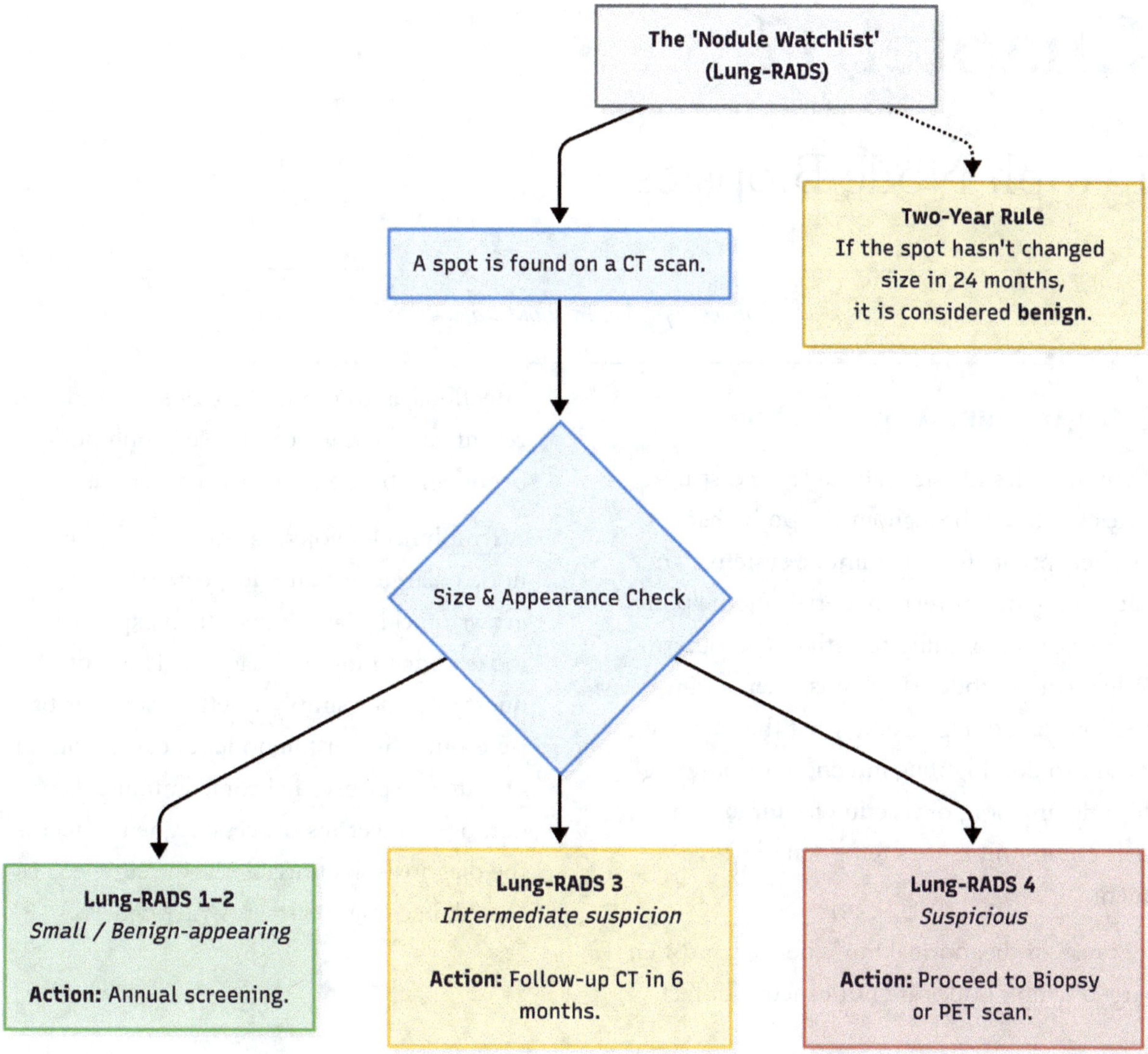
The 'Nodule Watchlist' (Lung-RADS)
A spot is found on a CT scan.
Two-Year Rule
If the spot hasn't changed size in 24 months, it is considered benign.
Size & Appearance Check
Lung-RADS 1–2
Small / Benign-appearing
Action: Annual screening.
Lung-RADS 3
Intermediate suspicion
Action: Follow-up CT in 6 months.
Lung-RADS 4
Suspicious
Action: Proceed to Biopsy or PET scan.

Chapter 17

Lymph Node Biopsies

Sorting Infection, Immunity, and Cancer

What It Is and Why It's Done

Lymph nodes are small, bean shaped structures scattered throughout the body that act as checkpoints for the immune system. They filter fluid, trap foreign material, and help immune cells communicate with one another. When lymph nodes swell, it is often a sign that they are doing exactly what they are meant to do. Fighting infection, responding to inflammation, or reacting to immune signals commonly causes temporary enlargement.

Because of this normal immune role, most enlarged lymph nodes are not cancer. In fact, infections, autoimmune conditions, and even recent vaccinations can cause lymph nodes to become noticeably larger for a period.

A lymph node biopsy is considered when a node enlarges for an unexpected reason, grows quickly, lasts longer than expected, or looks concerning on imaging. The central question is not simply whether cancer is present, but whether the node reflects a normal immune response, a chronic immune disorder, or a cancerous process. When cancer is the diagnosis, identifying the exact type is essential, because treatments vary widely.

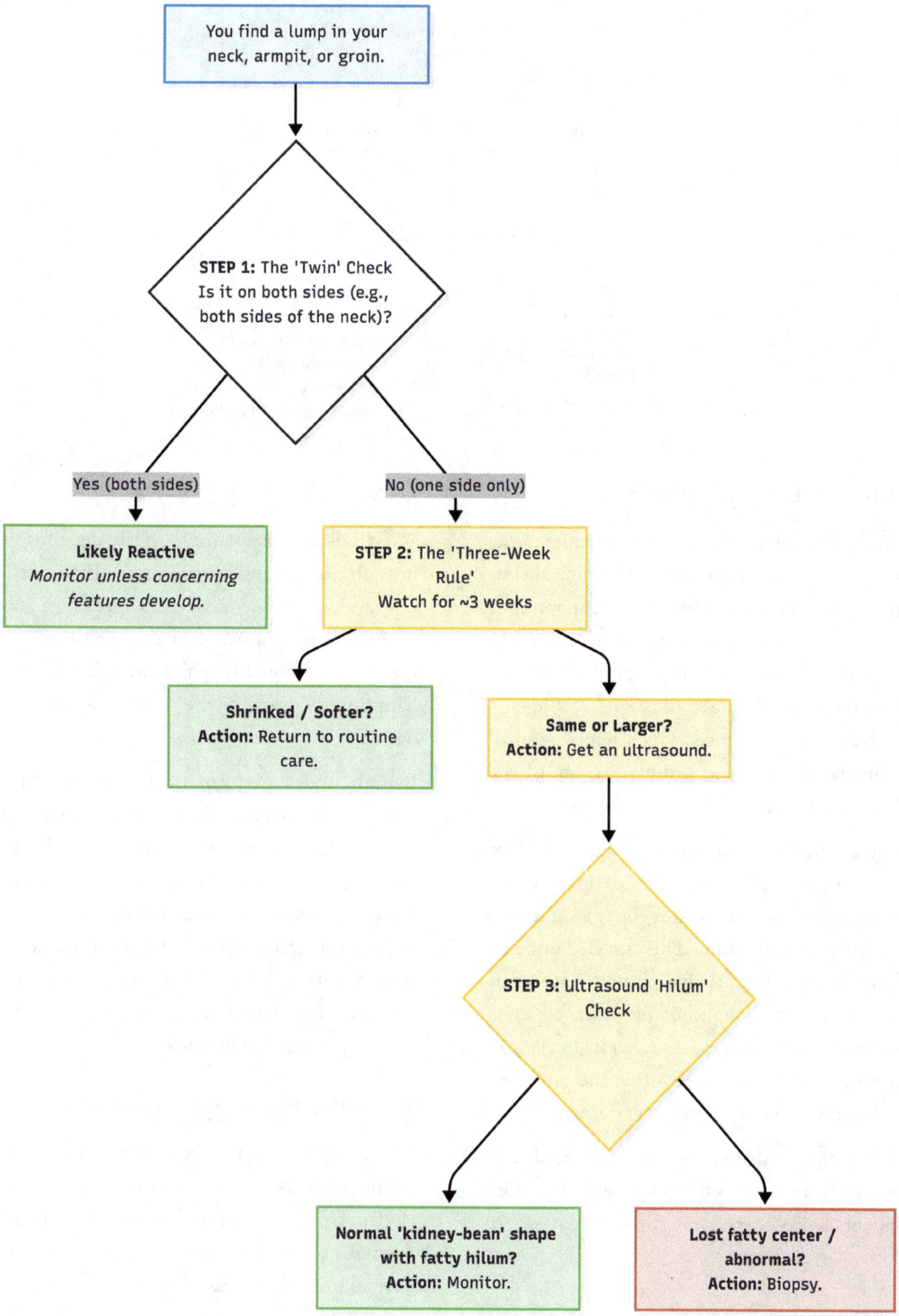
You find a lump in your neck, armpit, or groin.
STEP 1: The 'Twin' Check
Is it on both sides (e.g., both sides of the neck)?
Yes (both sides)
No (one side only)
Likely Reactive
Monitor unless concerning features develop.
STEP 2: The 'Three-Week Rule'
Watch for ~3 weeks
Shrinked / Softer?
Action: Return to routine care.
Same or Larger?
Action: Get an ultrasound.
STEP 3: Ultrasound 'Hilum' Check
Normal 'kidney-bean' shape with fatty hilum?
Action: Monitor.
Lost fatty center / abnormal?
Action: Biopsy.

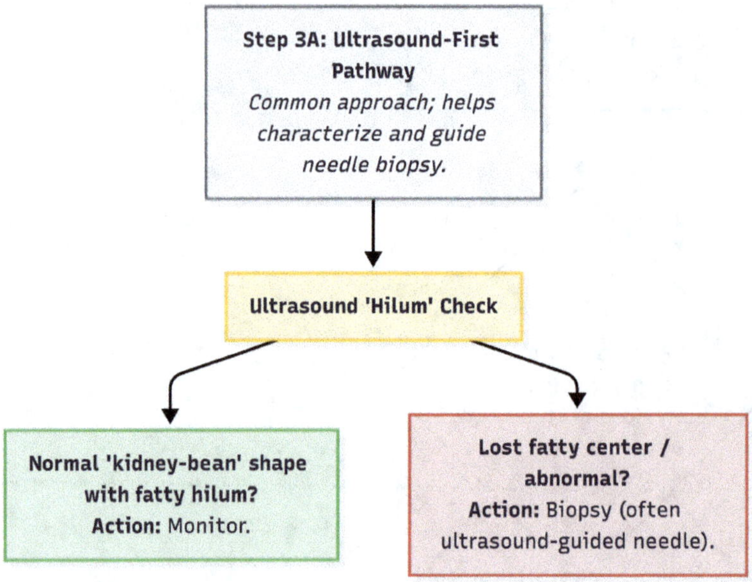

How the Biopsy Is Performed

There are several ways to sample a lymph node, and the approach depends on the clinical situation. In some cases, a fine needle aspiration is used. This involves a very thin needle, often guided by ultrasound, to collect individual cells from the node. In other situations, a core needle biopsy is performed, which removes small cylinders of tissue and preserves more of the node's structure.

When lymphoma is strongly suspected, or when prior needle biopsies do not provide enough information, a surgeon may remove the entire lymph node. This is called an excisional biopsy. Because lymph nodes are complex organs and lymphoma diagnosis depends on architecture as well as individual cells, removing the whole node is often the preferred first step when lymphoma is a concern.

Most lymph node biopsies are performed with local anesthesia, sometimes with light sedation. Patients typically go home the same day.

In the Pathology Laboratory

What reaches the pathology lab depends on how the biopsy was performed. Fine needle aspirations provide loose cells spread on glass slides. Core biopsies provide small pieces of tissue. Excisional biopsies provide an entire lymph node, allowing the most complete evaluation.

Lymph nodes perform many immune functions, so the tissue is often divided for multiple types of testing. Some is examined under the routine microscope to assess structure and cell patterns. Some may be sent for flow cytometry, a specialized test that analyzes immune cell populations in detail. Additional portions may be saved for special stains or genetic studies that help refine the diagnosis.

What the Pathologist Looks For

The first task is to determine whether the lymph node is reacting normally or showing evidence of a clonal process, meaning one abnormal group of cells has expanded beyond normal immune control. Many biopsies show reactive changes. These nodes may appear enlarged and busy under the microscope but remain well organized, reflecting responses to infections, autoimmune diseases, inflammation, or recent immune stimulation.

When cancer is present, it usually falls into one of two broad categories. One is lymphoma, a cancer that arises from immune cells and begins within the lymph nodes themselves. Lymphomas are divided into many specific types, broadly grouped as Hodgkin lymphoma and non Hodgkin lymphoma, each with distinct behaviors and treatments.

The second category is metastatic cancer. In these cases, cancer started elsewhere in the body and spread to the lymph node. Common sources include colon, breast, lung, skin (melanoma), and cancers of the head and neck. Distinguishing lymphoma from metastatic cancer is critical, because the treatment strategies are entirely different.

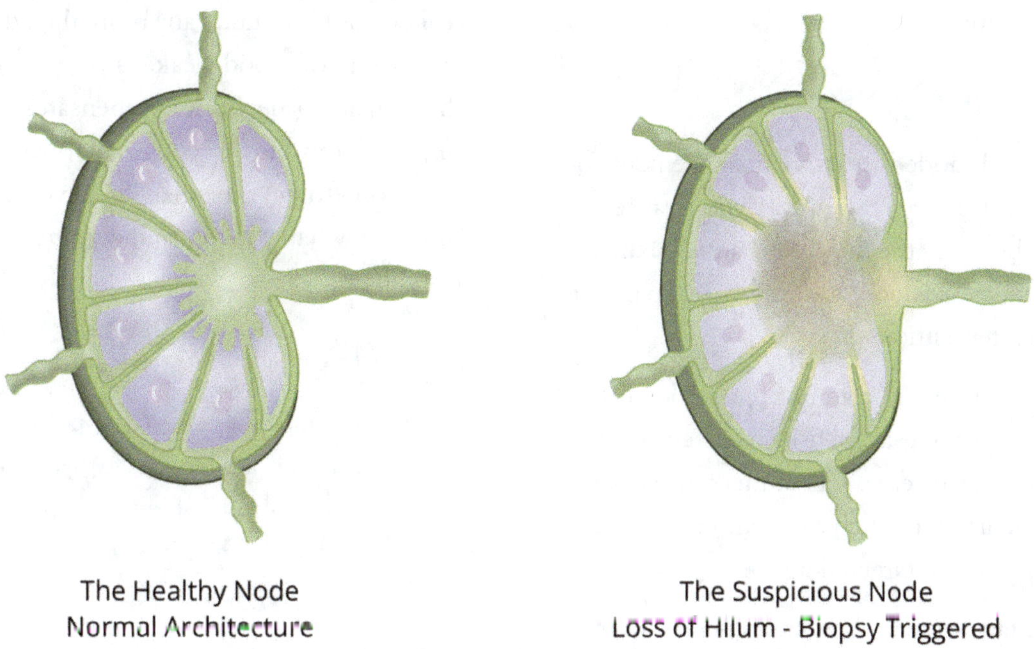

Figure 28. Illustration of lymph node showing normal architecture of hilum vs. loss of normal hilum architecture.

How Results Are Reported

Pathology reports often begin by stating whether the lymph node shows reactive changes or malignancy. A diagnosis of a reactive lymph node means that no cancer is identified and that the enlargement reflects immune activity rather than malignancy.

If lymphoma is diagnosed, the report names the specific type. This level of detail is essential, because treatment decisions depend on the exact subtype, not simply the presence of lymphoma. Some lymphomas grow slowly and may initially be observed, while others require prompt treatment.

When metastatic cancer is found, the report typically describes the type of cancer and may suggest the most likely site of origin. Special markers (immunohistochemical stains) are often used to help pinpoint where the cancer began.

Occasionally, a report uses terms such as atypical or suspicious. This usually means the sample was limited or showed unusual features that did not meet full criteria for a definitive diagnosis. In these situations, additional tissue, often a full lymph node, is recommended to reach certainty.

What Happens Next

If the lymph node is reactive, management focuses on treating the underlying cause or simply observing the node over time. Many reactive nodes gradually return to normal size without intervention.

When lymphoma is diagnosed, additional imaging and blood tests are used to determine the extent of the disease. Treatment usually involves medications such as chemotherapy, immunotherapy, or targeted agents.

If metastatic cancer is identified, the biopsy helps confirm the primary cancer and guides systemic treatment aimed at the whole body. In many cases, lymph node biopsy leads towards medical therapies that address disease wherever it is present.

Common Fears and Reassurances

When a patient feels a swollen lymph node in their neck for the first time, they often go straight to the worst possibility in their head. I understand. A node you can feel under the skin is a strange and unwelcome new shape. But by the time most of those nodes reach my microscope, the story they tell is far more ordinary. Reactive hyperplasia from a recent viral infection. A post-vaccination response. An old throat irritation the body decided to mount a defense against. The node was doing its job.

Lymphoma and metastatic cancer do occur, and identifying them is the reason we biopsy nodes that grow, persist, or look wrong on imaging. But the human body carries hundreds of lymph nodes spread along every major drainage path. Removing one for diagnosis does not weaken your immunity any more than donating a single cup of blood weakens your circulation. The remaining network compensates immediately, and the biopsy you went through provides something the imaging never could: a name for what your immune system was responding to.

Example

A young adult noticed a firm lymph node in the neck after a viral illness. After watchful waiting, a biopsy was performed and showed a reactive lymph node, and the swelling resolved over the following weeks without treatment.

In another case, a patient with night sweats and unintentional weight loss underwent removal of a lymph node. Pathology revealed Hodgkin lymphoma, allowing prompt treatment with an excellent long term outlook.

In a third situation, a small lymph node under the arm was biopsied and found to contain metastatic breast cancer. This discovery allowed systemic therapy to begin before more widespread disease developed.

What This Means for You

A lymph node biopsy is a tool for understanding why your immune system is signaling. It helps answer whether a node is reacting normally, involved by lymphoma, or affected by cancer that began elsewhere.

If a biopsy is recommended, it is reasonable to ask what the leading possibilities are, whether more tissue might be needed, and how the results will guide treatment. Most enlarged lymph nodes are benign, and when cancer is found, lymph node biopsies provide the essential roadmap for effective, targeted care rather than guesswork.

Questions to Ask Your Doctor During a Follow-up Appointment

Understanding the Why

1. Was the swelling caused by an infection, inflammation, or something else? (Sometimes nodes swell just because you had a recent cold or a scratch.)
2. Is this Reactive? (This is a common, friendly term that means the node is just reacting to something normal in your environment.)
3. What is the specific name of the cells found? (If the result is more serious, ask if it is a Lymphoma or if it is Metastatic, which means cancer cells that traveled from somewhere else.)

On the Result Details

1. Was the sample big enough to be sure? (Lymph nodes are complex; sometimes a tiny needle doesn't see the whole picture, and a larger sample is needed.)

Next Steps

1. Do I need more scans, like a PET or CT scan? (This helps see if other lymph nodes in the body are also activated.)
2. Should I see a specialist, like a Hematologist or an Oncologist?
3. If it was just an infection, do I need a round of antibiotics to help it shrink?

Recommended Lymph Node Exam Protocol

Doctors follow a very specific wait and watch vs. act now protocol to ensure you aren't getting unnecessary procedures for simple, temporary swelling.

The Physical Map Protocol

The first step is a physical exam. Doctors look at three main things to decide if a node is suspicious:

- Size: Nodes smaller than 1 centimeter (about the size of a pea) are usually considered safe.
- Texture: A good node is soft and moves easily under the skin. A concerning node feels hard, fixed in place, or like a rubber ball.
- Pain: Interestingly, a painful node is often a good sign, it usually means it's fighting a normal infection. Painless, hard nodes are the ones that trigger the biopsy protocol.

The Three-Week Rule

This is the most common protocol used by primary care doctors:

- If a lymph node is swollen but you have no other symptoms (like fever or weight loss), the protocol is to wait 3 to 4 weeks.

- Most reactive nodes from a cold or virus will shrink on their own in this time. If the node stays large or keeps growing after a month, the biopsy protocol is triggered.

The Imaging Protocol (Ultrasound First)

- Before jumping to a biopsy, the doctor will often order an Ultrasound.
- The radiologist looks for the Hilum, the fatty center of the lymph node.
- Protocol: If the node has lost its normal kidney bean shape or the fatty center has disappeared, a biopsy is usually recommended immediately.

The Architecture Protocol (Choosing the Biopsy Type)

When it comes to lymph nodes, the type of biopsy matters:

- FNA (Fine Needle): Often used first to see if cancer from another organ (like the breast or lung) has spread to the node.
- Excisional (Whole Node Removal): If the doctor is looking for Lymphoma (cancer that starts in the immune system), the protocol usually requires taking the entire node. This is because the pathologist needs to see the architecture (the way the cells are arranged inside) to give a 100% certain answer.

Author Tip: The 'Three-Week' Waiting Room

The Power of Patience: Most reactive nodes caused by a virus begin to shrink within ~21 days.

If it's still there after a month, the biopsy becomes much more meaningful because the 'noise' of common infections has been ruled out.

Quick Summary

- Most enlarged lymph nodes are reactive — they are responding to infection, inflammation, or recent vaccination, not signaling cancer.
- The body has hundreds of lymph nodes; removing one does not weaken your immune system.
- A persistent, painless, hard, or growing node (especially one that loses its normal shape on ultrasound) is the kind that needs biopsy.
- When lymphoma is suspected, an entire node is usually removed because the diagnosis depends on the node's internal architecture, not just its cells.
- When cancer is found, the biopsy distinguishes lymphoma (cancer that starts in

the node) from metastasis (cancer that traveled there) — two completely different treatment paths.

Chapter 18

Bladder Biopsies

Understanding What Blood in the Urine Means

What It Is and Why It's Done

Finding blood in the urine can be alarming. For many people, it is the first visible sign that something in the bladder needs closer attention.

A bladder biopsy is performed to answer one essential question: what is happening in the bladder lining? Is the tissue simply irritated, showing early warning changes, or does it contain cancer, and if so, how serious is it?

How the Biopsy Is Performed

Bladder biopsies are performed during a short procedure called a cystoscopy. A thin camera is gently passed through the urethra into the bladder, allowing the urologist to directly inspect the bladder lining. This direct view is important, because bladder abnormalities are often visible rather than hidden deep within tissue.

If an area appears abnormal, small samples are taken for biopsy. When there is a visible growth, it is usually removed during the same procedure. This removal is called a transurethral resection of bladder tumor, commonly abbreviated as TURBT. The term sounds intimidating, but it simply means shaving away abnormal tissue through the scope. This approach treats the visible problem while also providing tissue for diagnosis.

Some centers use special blue light techniques that make flat or subtle abnormal areas easier to see. After the procedure, it is common to experience mild burning with urination, temporary blood in the urine, or the short term use of a catheter. These effects usually improve within a few days.

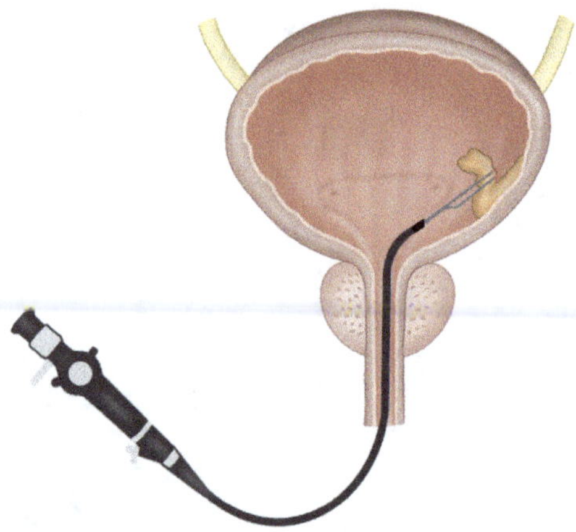

Figure 29. Trans urethral resection of bladder tumor (TURBT, i.e. removal of bladder tumor through cystoscope).

In the Pathology Laboratory

The tissue removed during biopsy or resection is sent to the pathology lab for examination. The most important task is determining how deep any abnormal cells extend into the bladder wall.

The bladder is made of layers. Some abnormalities stay confined to the surface lining. Others grow deeper and may reach the muscle layer. Knowing how far the cells have extended is the single most important factor in determining the seriousness of the condition and the appropriate treatment.

What the Pathologist Looks For

The first step is to determine whether the tissue shows non-cancerous changes such as inflammation, infection, or irritation. These are common causes of bleeding and are often related to infections, stones, or prior treatments rather than cancer.

When cancer is the diagnosis, several key questions follow. One is whether the cancer is limited to the surface or has begun to grow deeper. Tumors confined to the lining or just beneath it are called non muscle invasive and are the common types. Another question is whether the tumor has reached the bladder muscle. Once cancer involves the muscle, it behaves more aggressively and requires a different treatment approach. A third consideration is how aggressive the cancer cells appear under the microscope. Low grade tumors tend to grow slowly and recur locally, while high grade tumors have a higher risk of progression and spread.

An additional critical detail is whether bladder muscle is included in the biopsy specimen. If muscle is not present, the pathologist cannot be completely certain how deep the tumor extends. In that situation, another procedure may be recommended to ensure nothing more serious is missed.

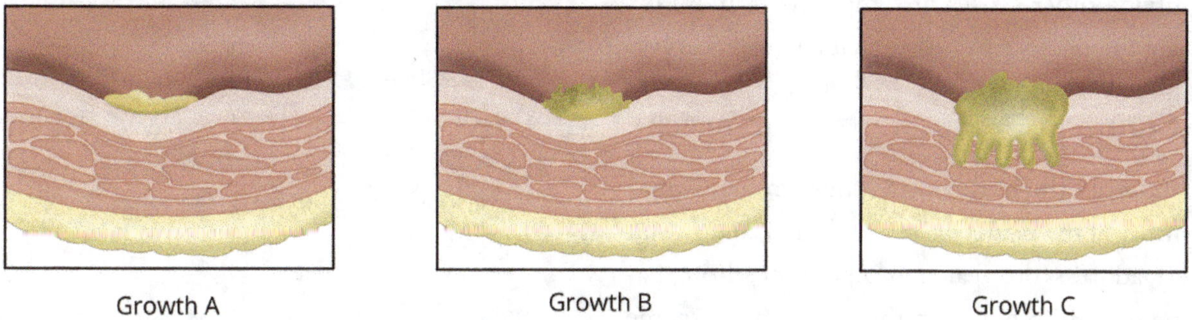

Figure 30. (A) Illustration of benign polyp; (B) early cancer; and (C) bladder cancer that involves the muscle layer of the bladder wall.

How Results Are Reported

Pathology reports use specific terms that guide treatment decisions. A report stating that no cancer is found means that benign changes explain the symptoms. A diagnosis of non muscle invasive bladder cancer indicates that the tumor is limited to the surface layers. Carcinoma in situ refers to flat, high grade cancer cells that remain on the surface but still require treatment because of their aggressive potential. Muscle invasive bladder cancer means the tumor has reached the muscle layer and calls for more intensive therapy.

These terms are not labels meant to frighten. They are tools your doctor uses to choose treatment that is appropriate to the actual risk, avoiding both undertreatment and unnecessary overtreatment.

What Happens Next

When bladder cancer is non muscle invasive, treatment often stays within the bladder. Many patients receive medication placed directly into the bladder to reduce the risk of recurrence. Because these tumors can come back, regular follow up cystoscopies are part of long term care and allow early detection if changes recur.

If the cancer has invaded the muscle, treatment usually involves a combination of approaches, such as chemotherapy, surgery, and sometimes radiation. Although this can sound overwhelming, decisions are made carefully and step by step, guided by strong evidence and tailored to the individual patient.

If no cancer is found, the focus shifts to identifying other causes of symptoms or monitoring the bladder to ensure that changes resolve.

Common Fears and Reassurances

Blood in the urine is the symptom that brings most of my bladder cases to the lab, and I want to address the fear it produces head-on. Patients who see pink in the toilet often assume the worst, and the worst is rarely the truth. Hematuria has many causes — urinary tract infections, kidney stones, blood thinners, vigorous exercise, even some foods. When it does turn out to be a tumor, the bladder is unusual among cancer sites in how often we catch the disease early, because the bleeding is too startling to ignore. People come in. We look.

The second fear I hear is that any bladder cancer diagnosis means losing the bladder. That picture is decades out of date. Most of the bladder cancers I signed out are non-muscle-invasive, meaning the disease is confined to the surface lining. These are typically treated by removing the visible tumor through a cystoscope and then using medication delivered directly into the bladder to lower the chance of recurrence. The bladder stays. The monitoring is regular, the long-term outcomes are good, and cystectomy — full removal — is reserved for the cancers that have grown into the muscle and demand it.

Example

One patient noticed painless blood in the urine and underwent cystoscopy. A small growth was found and removed during the same procedure. Pathology showed an early, surface level cancer. With treatment delivered directly into the bladder and routine follow up visits, the patient returned to normal life without further problems.

Another patient had a tumor that extended into the muscle layer. Because it was identified promptly, treatment began early, and the outcome was far better than it would have been if diagnosis had been delayed.

What This Means for You

A bladder biopsy is unusual among diagnostic procedures in that the urologist often sees the abnormality with their own eyes during cystoscopy, samples it in the same sitting, and may even remove the visible tumor entirely through the scope. By the time the slides reach my microscope, the question is rarely whether something was there; it is what the something turns out to be.

Most of the time the answer is good news. Inflammation, irritation from a stone or a recent infection, a small low-grade tumor confined to the surface lining that we now know how to treat with bladder-preserving therapy. Even when the result is more serious, the bladder is one of the few organs where regular cystoscopy lets us track changes over years and intervene early. Your role in this is straightforward: do not ignore blood in the urine, do not delay the follow-up scopes once you are in the surveillance pathway, and stay in conversation with your urology team. The system that brought you this far is designed to keep working as long as you stay inside it.

Questions to Ask Your Doctor During a Follow-up Appointment

Understanding the Why

1. Was the finding benign (non-cancerous) or malignant (cancerous)? (This is the first and most important distinction.)
2. If it is benign, is it an inflammatory condition?
3. Is this Reactive? (Much like lymph nodes, the bladder lining can react and thicken due to long-term irritation from kidney stones, catheters, or chronic UTIs.)
4. What caused the red patches or polyps you saw? (Are they simple inflammatory polyps or something that needs more attention?)

On the Result Details

1. What is the Grade and Stage? (If a growth was found, Grade tells you how aggressive the cells look, and Stage tells you how deep they go into the bladder wall.)
2. Does the pathology match my symptoms? (If you have significant pain or blood in your urine but the biopsy is normal, ask what else could be causing the issue.)
3. Was Muscle included in the sample? (For certain growths, the doctor needs to see the muscle layer to ensure the diagnosis is 100% accurate.)

Next Steps

1. Do I need Intravesical therapy? (This involves putting liquid medicine, either to fight cancer or to calm inflammation, directly into the bladder.)
2. Should I see a specialist for Pain Management? (If the result is a chronic inflammatory condition like Interstitial Cystitis, a specialized physical therapist or urologist may be the next step.)
3. When is my next Cystoscopy? (If the result was a benign polyp or a low-grade tumor, the bladder requires regular maintenance checks.)

Author Tip: The 'Muscle' Requirement

Ask about the Muscle: When you get your results, look for the phrase **'Muscularis propria present.'**

This is the pathologist's way of saying they had a deep enough sample to accurately determine the stage.

If the muscle wasn't captured in the 'shave,' your doctor may suggest a second look to be absolutely certain of the diagnosis.

Recommended Bladder Exam Protocol

The bladder protocol is designed to catch both aggressive diseases and chronic conditions that affect your quality of life.

The Physical & Visual Map Protocol

- The first step is a visual inspection. During a cystoscopy, doctors look for:
- Growth Type: Is it Papillary (looks like a tiny broccoli) or Sessile (flat against the wall)?
- Vascularity: Are there extra blood vessels or angry red patches?
- Capacity: How much fluid can the bladder hold before it becomes painful? (This is a key part of the protocol for chronic pain conditions.)

The Four-Week Rule for Irritation

- If a doctor sees a red, irritated patch in the bladder, they don't always biopsy it immediately.
- Initial Action: They may treat you for a hidden infection or ask you to remove bladder irritants (like tobacco) for a few weeks.
- The Trigger: If the patch is still there after 4 weeks, the protocol dictates a biopsy to ensure it isn't an early-stage flat growth (Carcinoma in Situ).

The Imaging Protocol (CT Urogram)

- If you have blood in your urine, the protocol often requires more than just a bladder biopsy.
- The Upper Tract Check: Doctors will order a specialized CT scan to look at the kidneys and the tubes (ureters) leading to the bladder. Why? The lining of the entire urinary system is the same. If the bladder is irritated, the protocol ensures the upstream parts are healthy too.

The Architecture Protocol (Choosing the Treatment)

The way the cells are arranged dictates the next step in the protocol:

- Benign Polyps: These are often sniped off during the biopsy. The protocol is usually one follow-up in 12 months to ensure no twins have grown back.

- Non-Invasive (Surface) Results: The protocol may involve a bladder wash with BCG (an immune activating therapy) or chemotherapy to prevent the cells from returning.
- Invasive Results: If cells have reached the muscularis propria (the muscle layer), the protocol shifts toward more intensive treatments, which may include surgery or radiation.

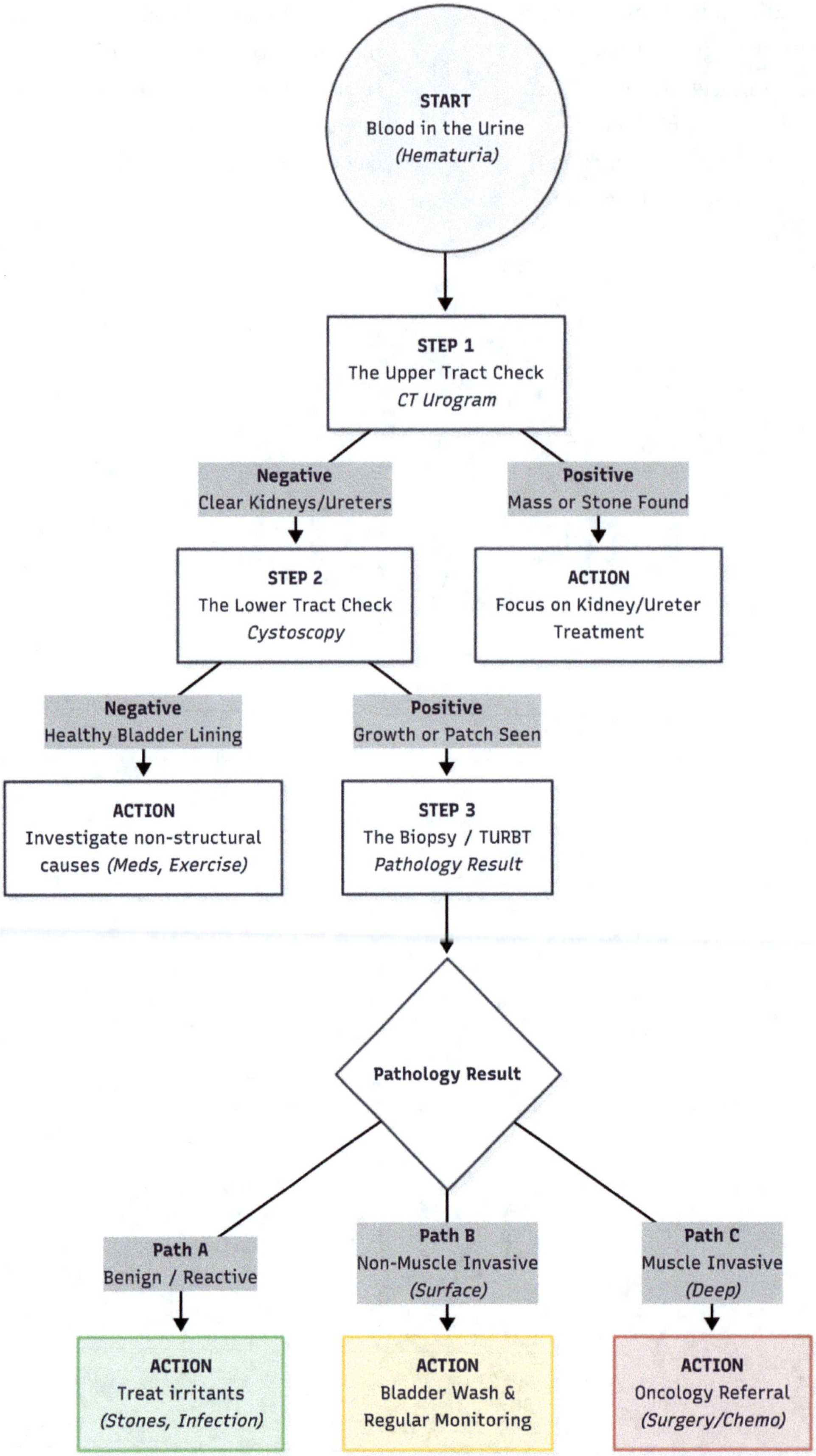
START
Blood in the Urine
(Hematuria)
STEP 1
The Upper Tract Check
CT Urogram
Negative
Clear Kidneys/Ureters
Positive
Mass or Stone Found
STEP 2
The Lower Tract Check
Cystoscopy
ACTION
Focus on Kidney/Ureter Treatment
Negative
Healthy Bladder Lining
Positive
Growth or Patch Seen
ACTION
Investigate non-structural causes (Meds, Exercise)
STEP 3
The Biopsy / TURBT
Pathology Result
Pathology Result
Path A
Benign / Reactive
Path B
Non-Muscle Invasive
(Surface)
Path C
Muscle Invasive
(Deep)
ACTION
Treat irritants
(Stones, Infection)
ACTION
Bladder Wash &
Regular Monitoring
ACTION
Oncology Referral
(Surgery/Chemo)

Quick Summary

- Blood in the urine is the most important early signal of bladder disease and should always be evaluated, even if it appears only once.
- Bladder biopsies are done during cystoscopy, which lets the urologist see and sample suspicious areas directly through a thin scope.
- The single most important question the pathologist answers is depth: has the cancer reached the bladder muscle? This determines everything that follows.
- Most bladder cancers are non-muscle-invasive and can be treated with bladder-preserving therapies (often medication delivered directly into the bladder).
- Bladder removal is a last resort, not a first step. Many cancers are controlled for years with localized treatment and routine monitoring.

Chapter 19

Kidney Biopsies

Two Different Questions, One Clear Answer

What It Is and Why It's Done

Kidney biopsies are performed for two distinct but equally important reasons. One reason is to understand medical kidney disease, meaning conditions that affect how the kidneys function. This situation often arises when blood or protein appears in the urine, when kidney function numbers such as creatinine begin to rise, or when a transplanted kidney is not working as expected.

The second reason for a kidney biopsy is to evaluate a mass seen on imaging. Some kidney masses are benign, some are cancerous, and others fall into a gray zone where careful monitoring may be the safest choice. In both settings, the biopsy serves the same purpose: it replaces educated guessing with specific information that directly shapes the treatment plan.

How the Biopsy Is Performed

Most kidney biopsies are performed using ultrasound guidance and a needle. You are positioned either on your stomach or, in the case of a transplanted kidney, on your back. The skin is cleaned and numbed, and a spring loaded needle quickly removes a few very small cores of tissue. The sensation is usually one of pressure rather than pain, and the sampling itself takes only seconds.

After the procedure, you are monitored closely, often for several hours, to watch for bleeding. This observation period is an important part of the process and is the reason the biopsy is usually done in a hospital or outpatient center rather than a clinic office. Most people go home the same day and are advised to avoid heavy lifting for a short time. If you take blood thinners, your care team provides specific instructions about when to stop and restart them to minimize risk of bleeding.

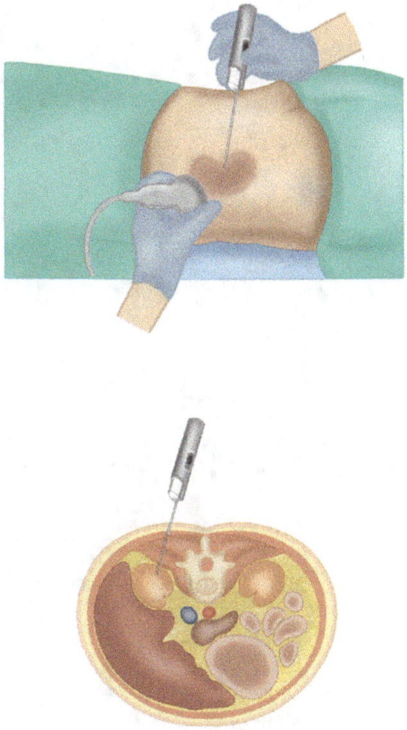

Figure 31. Transcutaneous kidney biopsy

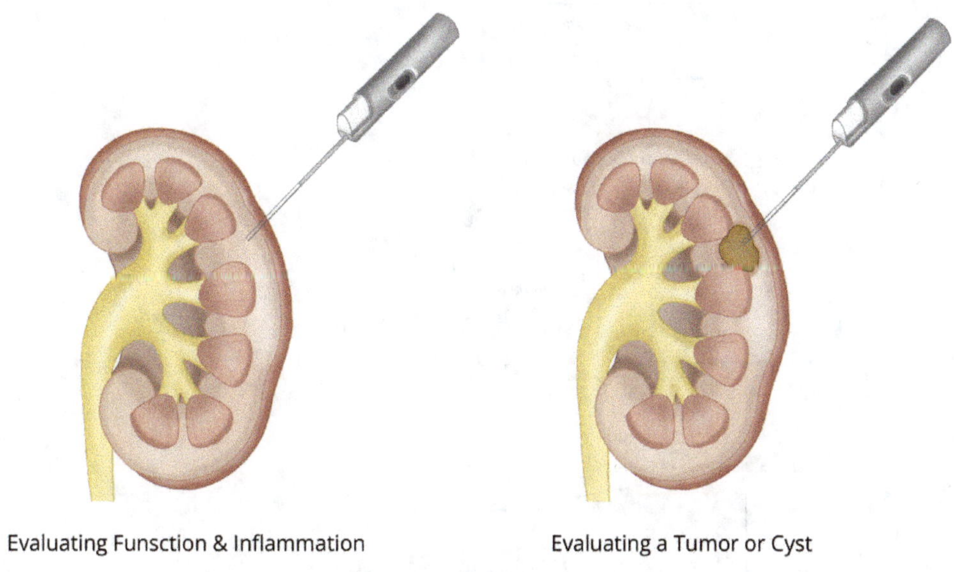

Figure 32. Kidney biopsy can be performed for evaluation of either the function of the kidney as a filtration organ or evaluation of a tumor arising in a kidney.

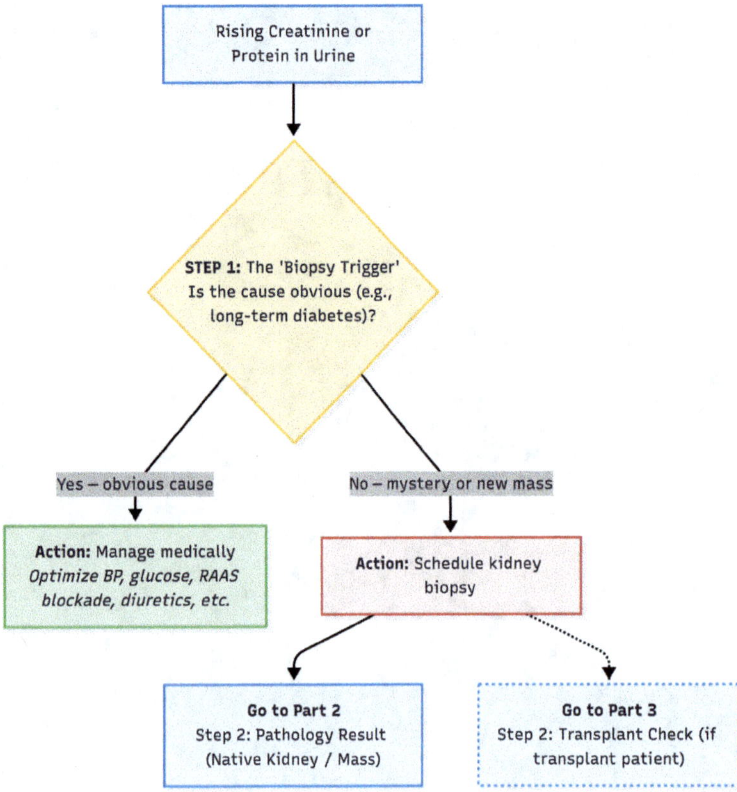
Rising Creatinine or Protein in Urine
STEP 1: The 'Biopsy Trigger' Is the cause obvious (e.g., long-term diabetes)?
Yes – obvious cause
No – mystery or new mass
Action: Manage medically Optimize BP, glucose, RAAS blockade, diuretics, etc.
Action: Schedule kidney biopsy
Go to Part 2 Step 2: Pathology Result (Native Kidney / Mass)
Go to Part 3 Step 2: Transplant Check (if transplant patient)

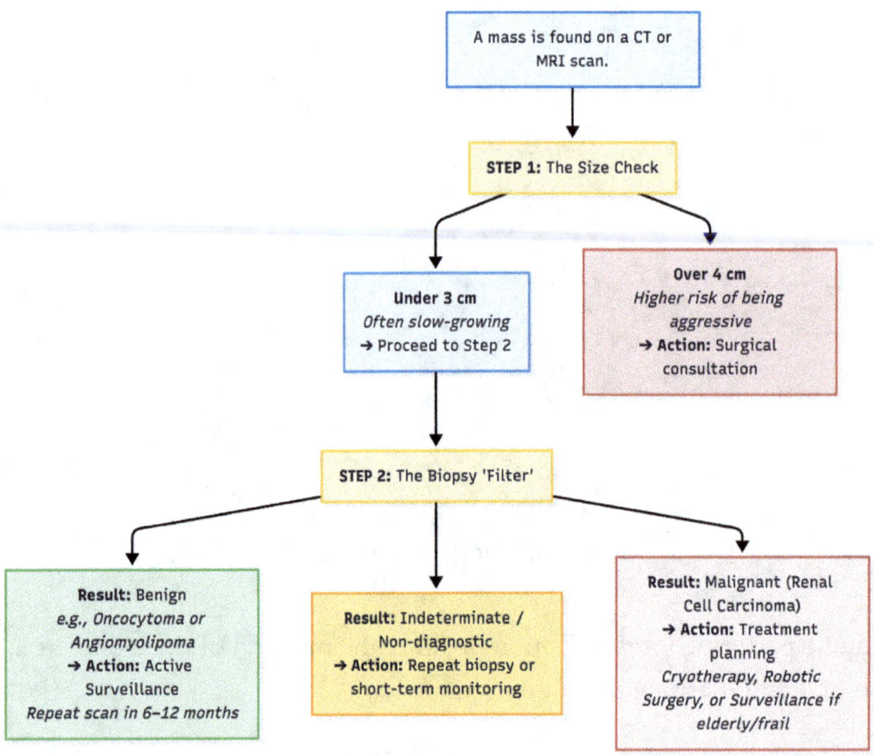
A mass is found on a CT or MRI scan.
STEP 1: The Size Check
Under 3 cm Often slow-growing → Proceed to Step 2
Over 4 cm Higher risk of being aggressive → Action: Surgical consultation
STEP 2: The Biopsy 'Filter'
Result: Benign e.g., Oncocytoma or Angiomyolipoma → Action: Active Surveillance Repeat scan in 6–12 months
Result: Indeterminate / Non-diagnostic → Action: Repeat biopsy or short-term monitoring
Result: Malignant (Renal Cell Carcinoma) → Action: Treatment planning Cryotherapy, Robotic Surgery, or Surveillance if elderly/frail

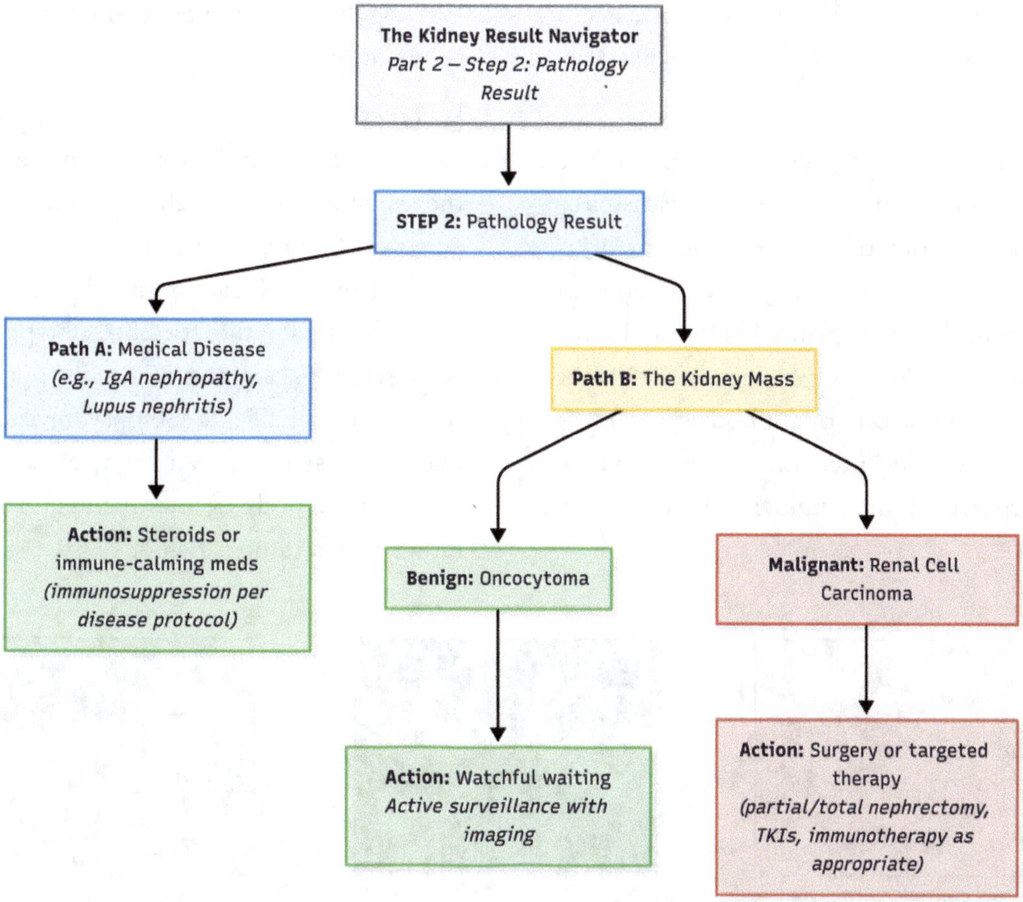

In the Pathology Laboratory

For medical kidney disease, the pathology lab usually receives two or three thin tissue cores. Each core is handled differently so the tissue can be examined using complementary techniques that together provide a complete picture of kidney health.

One portion is examined with the routine microscope, which shows the overall structure of the kidney, including scars, inflammation, and patterns of injury. Another portion is studied with special glowing stains that reveal whether immune proteins are depositing in the kidney's filtering units. A third portion may be examined with an electron microscope, which shows ultra fine details of the filters, called glomeruli, that cannot be seen any other way.

When the biopsy is performed for a kidney mass, the lab usually receives small cores that are processed for routine stains and, when needed, additional markers that help distinguish one tumor type from another.

What the Pathologist Looks For

In medical kidney disease, the pathologist examines all of the kidney's working parts: the tiny filters that clean the blood, the tubules that process fluid, the blood vessels that supply oxygen, and the supporting tissue between them. The goal is to recognize patterns that explain the patient's symptoms. These patterns may include inflammation, immune deposits, swelling, scarring, or injury caused by medications or toxins.

Common diagnoses include conditions such as IgA nephropathy, minimal change disease, focal segmental glomerulosclerosis, membranous nephropathy, diabetic kidney disease, and lupus nephritis. In transplanted kidneys, the focus shifts to identifying rejection, whether driven by immune cells or antibodies, as well as medication toxicity, infection such as BK virus, or recurrence of the original kidney disease. Delving deeper into these entities is beyond the scope of this book.

When evaluating a kidney mass, the task is different. The pathologist determines whether the lesion is benign (such as an oncocytoma or angiomyolipoma) or malignant, most often a form of renal cell carcinoma. If cancer is present, identifying the specific subtype matters because prognosis and treatment options differ. Occasionally, the biopsy reveals that a mass represents spread from a cancer elsewhere in the body or an inflammatory process rather than a tumor at all.

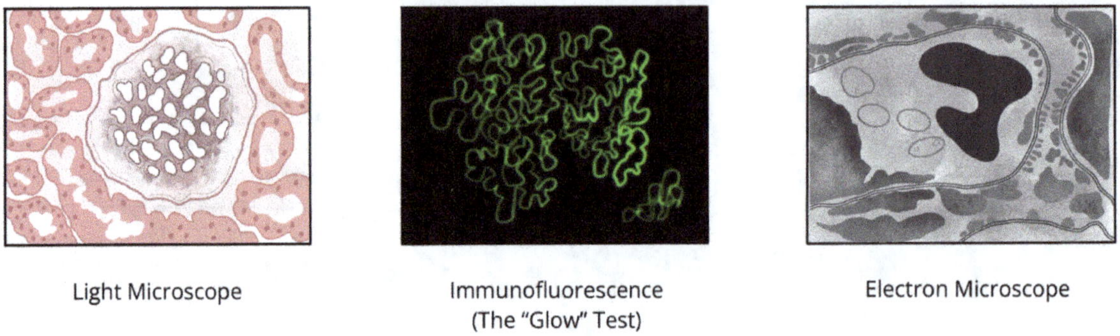

Figure 33. Microscopic appearance of the kidney filtration system.

How Results Are Reported

For medical kidney disease, the pathology report explains the diagnosis and includes practical details that help guide treatment. The report often notes how many filters were present in the sample, whether there is active inflammation, and how much permanent scarring is present. Scarring is commonly described using the terms interstitial fibrosis and tubular atrophy, often abbreviated as IFTA. These details help predict how much kidney function can recover and which therapies are likely to be helpful.

In transplant biopsies, reports use standardized language to grade rejection and describe specific findings that point toward immune injury. Certain stains provide clues about antibody involvement, which directly influences treatment choices.

For kidney masses, the report clearly states whether the lesion is benign or cancerous and names the specific type. When the diagnosis requires confirmation, additional stains and molecular tests are added so the urologist or nephrologist has what they need to choose the next step.

What Happens Next

For medical kidney disease, biopsy results guide targeted therapy. Some conditions respond well to steroids or other medications that calm the immune system, while others are managed with blood pressure control, reduction of urine protein, or changes to medications that may be stressing the kidneys. In transplant patients, biopsy findings allow doctors to tailor anti rejection treatment and adjust immune suppression carefully to protect the graft.

For a kidney mass, the results help determine whether watchful waiting, minimally invasive treatment, surgery, or medication is the best option. Benign lesions may be followed with periodic imaging, while cancers are managed based on their size, type, and whether they have spread.

Common Fears and Reassurances

The kidneys are stubbornly vascular organs. They filter every drop of blood in your body every few minutes, which is why bleeding is the complication patients ask about most. The honest answer is that some bleeding is common after a kidney biopsy, and almost all of it is microscopic and self-limited. You will lie flat for a few hours afterward not because the team expects a problem, but because pressure and rest are how the kidney seals the needle track on its own. Serious bleeding requiring intervention is uncommon, particularly with image guidance, and the post-procedure observation period exists specifically to catch it early on the rare occasion it occurs.

The other concern is the sample itself. A medical kidney biopsy needs a minimum number of filtering units, the glomeruli, to give a confident diagnosis. When I receive the cores, the first thing I do is count them. If the count is too low — sometimes a few millimeters of cortex away from a confident answer — I will say so, and the team will plan accordingly. The biopsy is not pass or fail. It is information about the kidney; sometimes the information includes "we need a bit more tissue."

Example

A young adult developed sudden leg swelling and was found to have very high levels of protein in the urine. A kidney biopsy showed minimal change disease, a condition that often responds quickly to steroid treatment. Within weeks, the protein levels normalized and symptoms improved.

In another case, a kidney transplant recipient experienced a gradual rise in creatinine. Biopsy revealed antibody mediated rejection. Prompt, targeted therapy brought kidney function back toward normalcy and helped preserve the transplant.

In a third situation, a patient with a small kidney mass underwent biopsy that showed an oncocytoma, a benign tumor. With that in mind, the patient chose active surveillance and avoided unnecessary surgery.

> **Author Tip: The 'Incidentaloma'**
>
> **The Discovery Dilemma:** Many kidney masses are now found *incidentally*—discovered while you were getting a scan for a completely different reason, such as a stomach ache or a back injury.
>
> Because we are finding them so much earlier, we have the luxury of using a biopsy to safely 'wait and watch' many of these small spots rather than rushing into the operating room.

What This Means for You

A kidney biopsy is often the definitive path to confirmation of a medical condition. You can expect a carefully planned, image guided procedure, a period of observation afterward, and results that directly influence your care.

It is reasonable to ask what the biopsy showed, whether there is active inflammation or mostly scarring, and how the findings affect treatment options. If you have a transplant, asking what type of rejection is present and how it is treated can be especially helpful. If a mass is involved, understanding whether it is benign or cancerous and what choices that opens up allows you to participate fully in decision making.

With those answers, the next step shifts from guessing to executing. For medical kidney disease, the biopsy points toward a specific medication or a specific reason to back off one. For a kidney mass, it tells the urologist whether the lesion can be watched, resected, or treated with focal ablation. The biopsy does not just describe; it directs.

Questions to Ask Your Doctor During a Follow-up Appointment

Understanding the Results

1. What is the name of my kidney problem? (For example: IgA Nephropathy, Lupus-related kidney inflammation, or Minimal Change Disease.)
2. Did my biopsy show active changes or chronic changes? Active means there is current inflammation that treatment can calm down. Chronic means there is older, permanent scarring. This helps you understand what can still improve.
3. How many kidney filters were in the biopsy sample? A good biopsy usually needs at least 10 filters (glomeruli) to get a clear picture of what's going on.

On Treatment and Lifestyle

1. Will I need medicines that calm the immune system, like steroids? Many kidney diseases happen because the immune system becomes overactive.
2. Do my blood pressure goals need to be lower now? Kidneys are very sensitive to blood pressure, so the target number may become stricter.
3. Should I change the way I eat? Ask about protein, salt, and potassium, your doctor may want you to adjust these based on your results.

4. Could this condition come back after a transplant or affect my other kidney? (Ask only if relevant)

Future Monitoring

1. What number or test are we going to follow to see how I'm doing? (For example: protein in my urine or my eGFR.)
2. Do I need regular visits with a Nephrologist?

Recommended Kidney Exam Protocol

Kidney health is checked using a Triple-Test approach: blood tests, urine tests, and sometimes a tissue sample. This gives the full picture.

The Screening Duo (Blood & Urine)

The basic starting point for kidney care includes two simple tests:

- eGFR (Estimated Glomerular Filtration Rate): A blood test that measures how well your kidneys clean your blood.
- UACR (Urine Albumin-to-Creatinine Ratio): A urine test that checks if protein is leaking out. Healthy kidneys normally keep protein in the bloodstream, if it shows up in urine, the filters may be damaged.

The Biopsy Trigger

A biopsy isn't needed for everyone. Doctors usually consider one when:

- Kidney function drops suddenly without a clear reason.
- There is a large amount of protein in the urine that can't be easily explained (like from diabetes).
- The urine shows signs of active glomeruli injury/process, such as dysmorphic (oddly shaped) red blood cells.
- There is a mass or tumor detected by imaging studies.

Post-Biopsy Safety Protocol

Since kidneys have a strong blood flow, safety after a biopsy is very important:

- The Flat Rule: You'll need to lie flat for 4 - 6 hours to reduce bleeding risk.
- The Pulse Check: Your vital signs (blood pressure and heart rate) will be checked often to ensure there's no internal bleeding.
- Hydration: You'll be encouraged to drink plenty of fluids to help the kidneys recover.
- The Lifting Limit: You shouldn't lift anything heavier than a gallon of milk for 1 - 2 weeks while the kidney heals.

Quick Summary

- A kidney biopsy answers two very different questions: how is the kidney functioning, or what is this mass on imaging.
- For functional disease, the sample is examined three ways (light microscopy, immune-protein stains, and electron microscopy) to identify the specific pattern of injury or inflammation.
- For a mass, the biopsy distinguishes benign tumors (like oncocytoma) from

cancer (most often renal cell carcinoma) and may help patients avoid unnecessary surgery.

- Bleeding is the main risk and is usually minor; you'll lie flat for several hours afterward and avoid heavy lifting for one to two weeks.
- The report often distinguishes active inflammation (which treatment can reverse) from chronic scarring (which is permanent) — both numbers shape your treatment plan.

Chapter 20

Liver Biopsy

Understanding What a Liver Mass Really Means

What It Is and Why It's Done

A mass in the liver can represent many different conditions. Some are completely benign. Others are primary liver cancers. Many turn out to be cancer that has spread from another organ, such as the colon, pancreas, breast, or lung. Because these possibilities can look similar on scans, imaging alone is often not enough.

A liver biopsy provides a definitive answer. Knowing exactly what a liver mass represents is essential, because treatment strategies differ dramatically depending on whether the tumor started in the liver or arrived there from elsewhere.

How the Biopsy Is Performed

Most liver biopsies are performed using ultrasound or CT guidance. A thin needle is passed through the skin into the liver to collect small tissue samples. The path is carefully chosen to avoid major blood vessels and nearby organs.

When bleeding risk is higher, the biopsy may be performed through a vein in the neck. In this approach, the needle reaches the liver from inside the blood vessels rather than through the abdominal wall, improving safety. After the procedure, patients are observed briefly and usually return home the same day.

What the Pathologist Looks For

The pathology lab receives tiny cores of liver tissue. Despite their small size, these samples are often sufficient to determine the nature of the lesion and to run additional tests. If there is underlying liver disease, such as cirrhosis or fatty liver, that information can be assessed at the same time and included in the report

The central question is whether the tumor began in the liver or represents metastatic disease. Primary liver cancers have distinct features that differ from tumors that spread from other organs. Special stains and tests help the pathologist make this distinction with confidence.

If cancer is present, additional testing may identify molecular features that influence treatment options, including eligibility for targeted therapies or clinical trials.

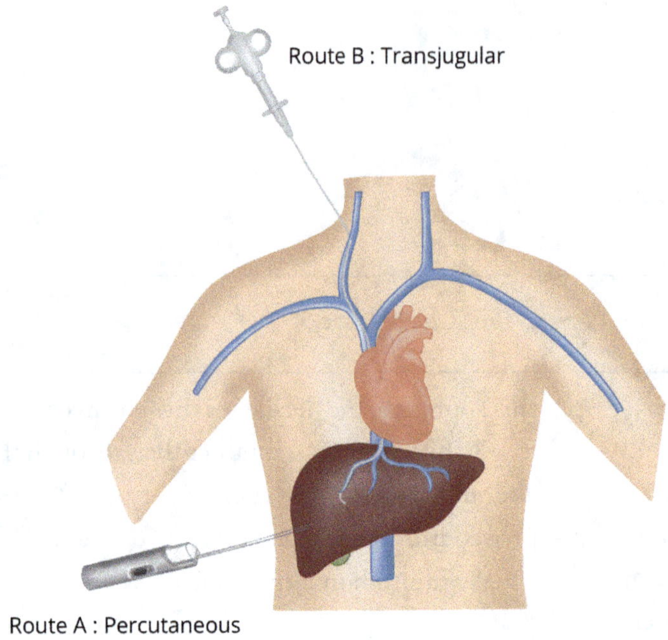

Figure 34. Illustration of approaches to liver biopsy. Percutaneous (A) and through the transjugular vein (B)

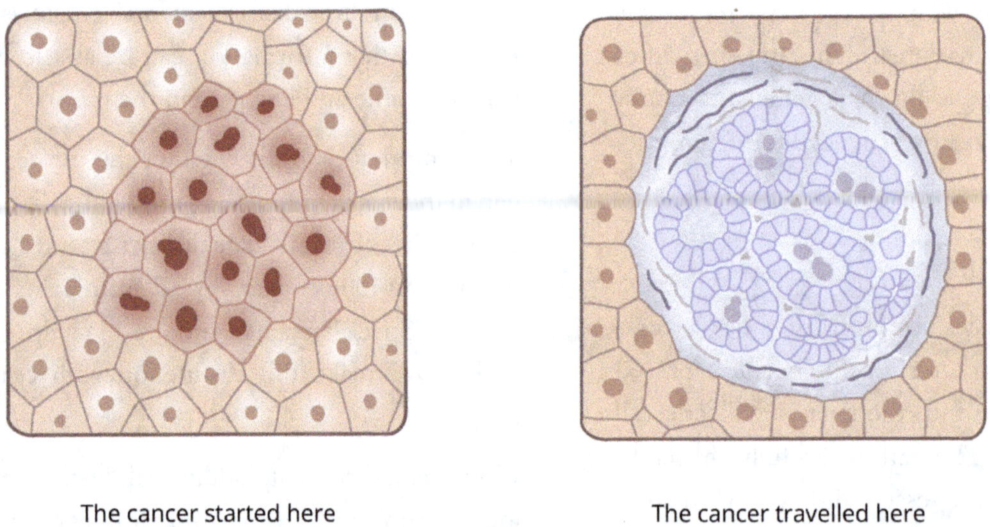

Figure 35. Illustration of appearance of liver tumor under the microscope. Primary liver cancer (left) and metastatic cancer to the liver from the colon (right).

How Results Are Reported

Liver biopsy reports aim to be direct and clear. Diagnoses may include such as hepatocellular carcinoma, cholangiocarcinoma (bild duct cancer), metastatic cancer to the liver, or benign tumor. When relevant, the report also includes information that helps guide treatment selection.

What Happens Next

Once the diagnosis is established, your care team integrates the biopsy findings with imaging, liver function, and overall health. Treatment may involve surgery, localized liver therapies, systemic medications, or supportive care aimed at preserving liver health. The biopsy ensures that therapy is matched to the true diagnosis rather than assumptions based on imaging alone.

Common Fears and Reassurances

The liver receives roughly a quarter of the body's cardiac output every minute, and that fact is the source of the question I am most often asked: is it safe to put a needle into it? In practice, the answer for the great majority of patients is yes. The radiologist uses ultrasound or CT to choose a path that avoids the major vessels, the bile ducts, and the gallbladder. The core itself is a thin cylinder, no thicker than a piece of spaghetti.

For patients whose blood does not clot normally, or whose anatomy makes the percutaneous route risky, there is an alternative: the transjugular approach. The needle enters through a vein in the neck and reaches the liver from inside its own venous drainage, so any bleeding stays where it belongs. When that approach lands a core on my desk, it is functionally identical to the cores I see from the more familiar through-the-skin route, and the underlying disease tells me the same story under the microscope.

What This Means for You

A liver biopsy determines what a liver mass truly represents and guides treatment decisions that can significantly affect outcomes. Even a very small sample can lead to the right care at the right time.

Author Tip: The 'Fatty' Reversal

A Resilient Organ: Unlike many other organs, the liver is a master of regeneration.

If your biopsy shows **'Steatosis'** (fatty liver) but only low levels of **'Fibrosis'** (scarring), lifestyle changes – including improvements in **diet** and reductions in **alcohol intake** – can actually reverse the damage.

It's one of the rare times a biopsy can show a clear path back to a completely healthy liver.

Questions to Ask Your Doctor During a Follow-up Appointment

Understanding the Results

1. What is the specific diagnosis? (e.g., Is it Non-Alcoholic Fatty Liver Disease (NAFLD), Hepatitis, or Autoimmune Liver Disease?)
2. If there is fibrosis, what is the Stage of fibrosis (scarring)? (Liver health is often graded on a scale from F0 to F4. F0 means no scarring, while F4 represents cirrhosis.)
3. What is the Grade of activity? (This measures how much active inflammation is happening in the liver right now.)

On Treatment and Management

1. Is the damage reversible? (The liver has a remarkable ability to heal if the underlying cause is addressed early.)
2. Do I need to change my medications? (Some common medications are processed by the liver and may need to be adjusted.)
3. Are there specific dietary changes I should make immediately?

Future Monitoring

1. How often will we repeat blood tests or imaging?
2. Do I need to be screened for liver cancer? (This is a standard protocol for patients with significant scarring.)

Recommended Liver Exam Protocol

Liver health is managed through a protocol of Screen, Grade, and Monitor. Because liver disease is often silent (causing no symptoms until it is advanced), these steps are critical.

The First-Line Screening

Most liver protocols begin with routine blood work called Liver Function Tests (LFTs). If enzymes like ALT or AST are persistently elevated, the protocol triggers:

- An Ultrasound: To look for physical changes like a fatty appearance or a change in liver size.
- Non-Invasive Fibrosis Testing: Tools like FibroScan (a specialized ultrasound that measures liver stiffness) are often used before a biopsy to see if significant scarring is present.

The Cirrhosis Surveillance Protocol

If a biopsy or FibroScan confirms Cirrhosis (F4 scarring), the protocol shifts to intensive surveillance for cancer. This is known as HCC Surveillance (Hepatocellular Carcinoma):

- Abdominal Ultrasound: Every 6 months.
- AFP Blood Test: Every 6 months to check for protein markers associated with liver cancer.

The Silent Fatty Liver Protocol (MASLD)

Because fatty liver disease is becoming more common, especially in people with diabetes or high cholesterol, doctors now follow a specific checklist of steps to help protect liver health. These steps include:

1. Annual LFTs: To monitor for inflammation.
2. Weight Management: The primary treatment protocol is a gradual reduction in body weight, which can often

melt fat out of the liver cells and reverse early-stage damage.

Post-Biopsy Safety Protocol

The liver is very rich in blood vessels, so the protocol after a biopsy focuses on preventing bleeding:

- Positioning: You will likely be asked to lie on your right side for 1 - 2 hours after the procedure to apply pressure to the biopsy site.
- Observation: Your blood pressure and heart rate will be monitored for several hours before you are released.
- Activity Restriction: Most protocols require avoiding heavy lifting or vigorous exercise for 5 to 7 days.

Quick Summary

- A liver biopsy answers what a liver mass or unexplained liver disease actually is — many possibilities look similar on imaging.
- The most important question for a tumor is origin: did it start in the liver, or did it spread there from another organ? Treatment is completely different.
- When safety requires it, the biopsy can be done through a vein in the neck (transjugular) rather than through the abdominal wall, reducing bleeding risk.
- Fatty liver, hepatitis, and early scarring are often reversible if caught and treated early; the biopsy can grade how much damage exists and how much active inflammation remains.
- Patients with cirrhosis need lifelong cancer surveillance: an abdominal ultrasound and AFP blood test every six months.

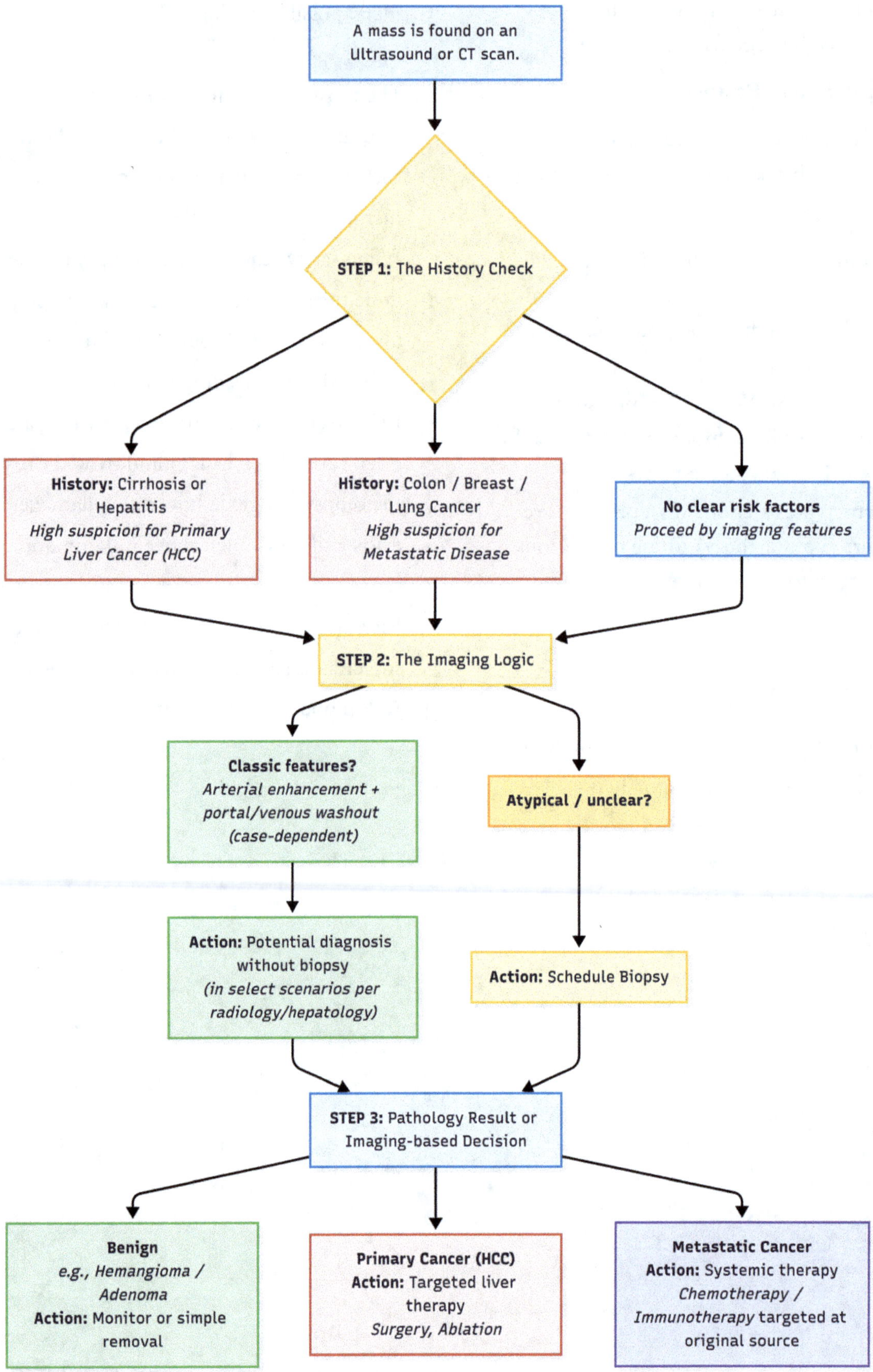
A mass is found on an Ultrasound or CT scan.
STEP 1: The History Check
History: Cirrhosis or Hepatitis
High suspicion for Primary Liver Cancer (HCC)
History: Colon / Breast / Lung Cancer
High suspicion for Metastatic Disease
No clear risk factors
Proceed by imaging features
STEP 2: The Imaging Logic
Classic features?
Arterial enhancement + portal/venous washout (case-dependent)
Atypical / unclear?
Action: Potential diagnosis without biopsy
(in select scenarios per radiology/hepatology)
Action: Schedule Biopsy
STEP 3: Pathology Result or Imaging-based Decision
Benign
e.g., Hemangioma / Adenoma
Action: Monitor or simple removal
Primary Cancer (HCC)
Action: Targeted liver therapy
Surgery, Ablation
Metastatic Cancer
Action: Systemic therapy
Chemotherapy / Immunotherapy targeted at original source

Chapter 21

Bone Marrow Biopsies

Understanding the Body's Blood Factory

What It Is and Why It's Done

Bone marrow is where your blood is made. Inside the soft center of certain bones, most commonly the back of the hip, your body continuously produces red blood cells that carry oxygen, white blood cells that fight infection, and platelets that help control bleeding. This process runs quietly in the background every day, adjusting to illness, stress, and recovery without you ever noticing.

When blood counts become abnormal or an illness affects the blood in a way that cannot be explained by routine tests, a bone marrow biopsy helps answer a crucial question. Is the marrow working normally, or has something disrupted the blood making process?

Because it looks directly at where blood cells are produced, a bone marrow biopsy is not ordered lightly. It is used when blood tests alone cannot fully explain what is happening and when understanding the marrow itself is essential to choosing the right next step.

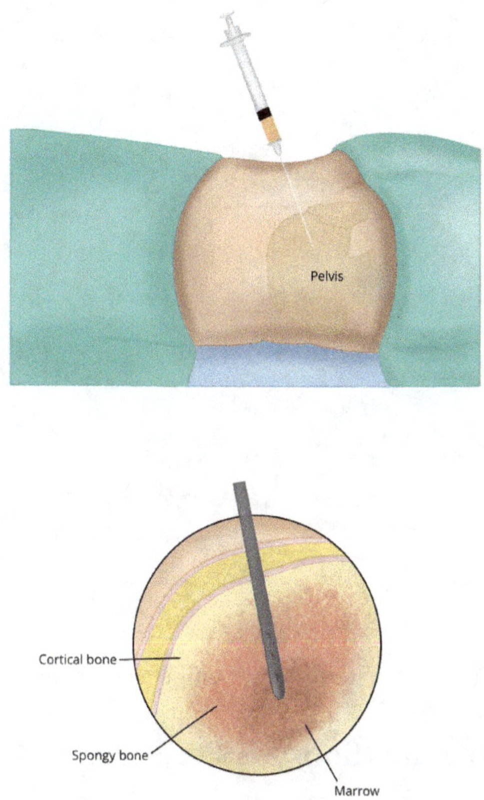

Figure 36. Bone marrow biopsy. Aspiration (top) and bone marrow biopsy (bottom).

Why a Bone Marrow Biopsy Is Done

Doctors recommend a bone marrow biopsy when blood counts are persistently too low or too high, when blood cells look abnormal under the microscope, or when symptoms such as ongoing fatigue, frequent infections, easy bruising or bleeding, fevers, or night sweats raise concern.

The biopsy helps determine whether a problem is temporary or long standing, reactive or primary, inherited or acquired, immune related, or due to a blood cancer. Common reasons for performing the test include evaluating unexplained anemia (low red blood cell and it's elements), low white blood cell counts, low platelets, suspected leukemia or lymphoma, plasma cell disorders such as multiple myeloma, and situations in which cancer from another part of the body may have spread to the marrow.

In short, the biopsy helps clarify whether the marrow is responding appropriately to stress or illness, or whether it has become the source of the problem itself.

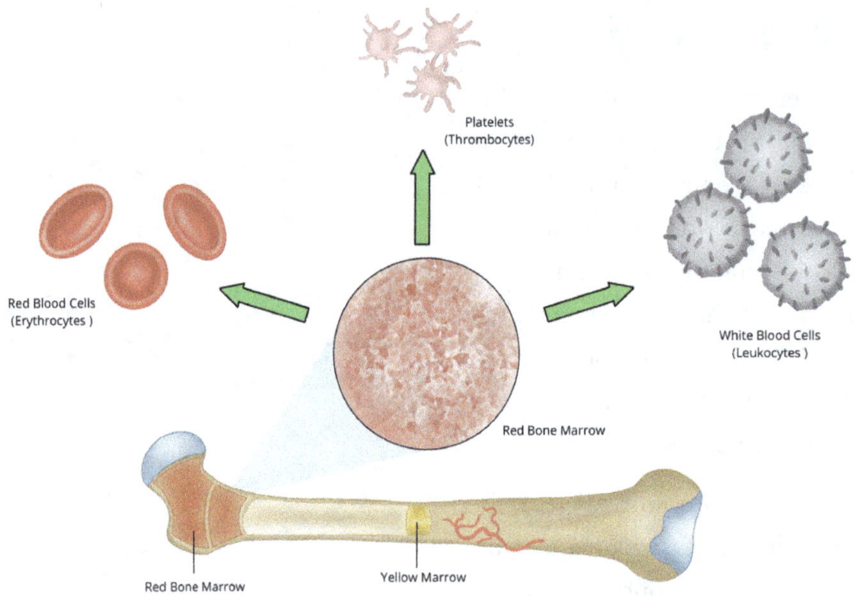

Figure 37. The different cell types produced from the bone marrow

How the Biopsy Is Performed

A bone marrow biopsy is usually performed from the back of the hip bone. After the skin and deeper tissues are numbed, the clinician first removes a small amount of liquid marrow, known as the aspirate. This step can cause a brief pulling or pressure sensation that lasts only a few seconds.

Next, a tiny core of solid marrow is removed. This is the biopsy portion of the procedure. The entire process typically takes about fifteen minutes. Most patients describe the discomfort as brief and manageable, even if it is unpleasant for a moment.

Afterward, you can usually go home the same day. Soreness at the biopsy site is common but typically fades over several days and can be managed with simple measures.

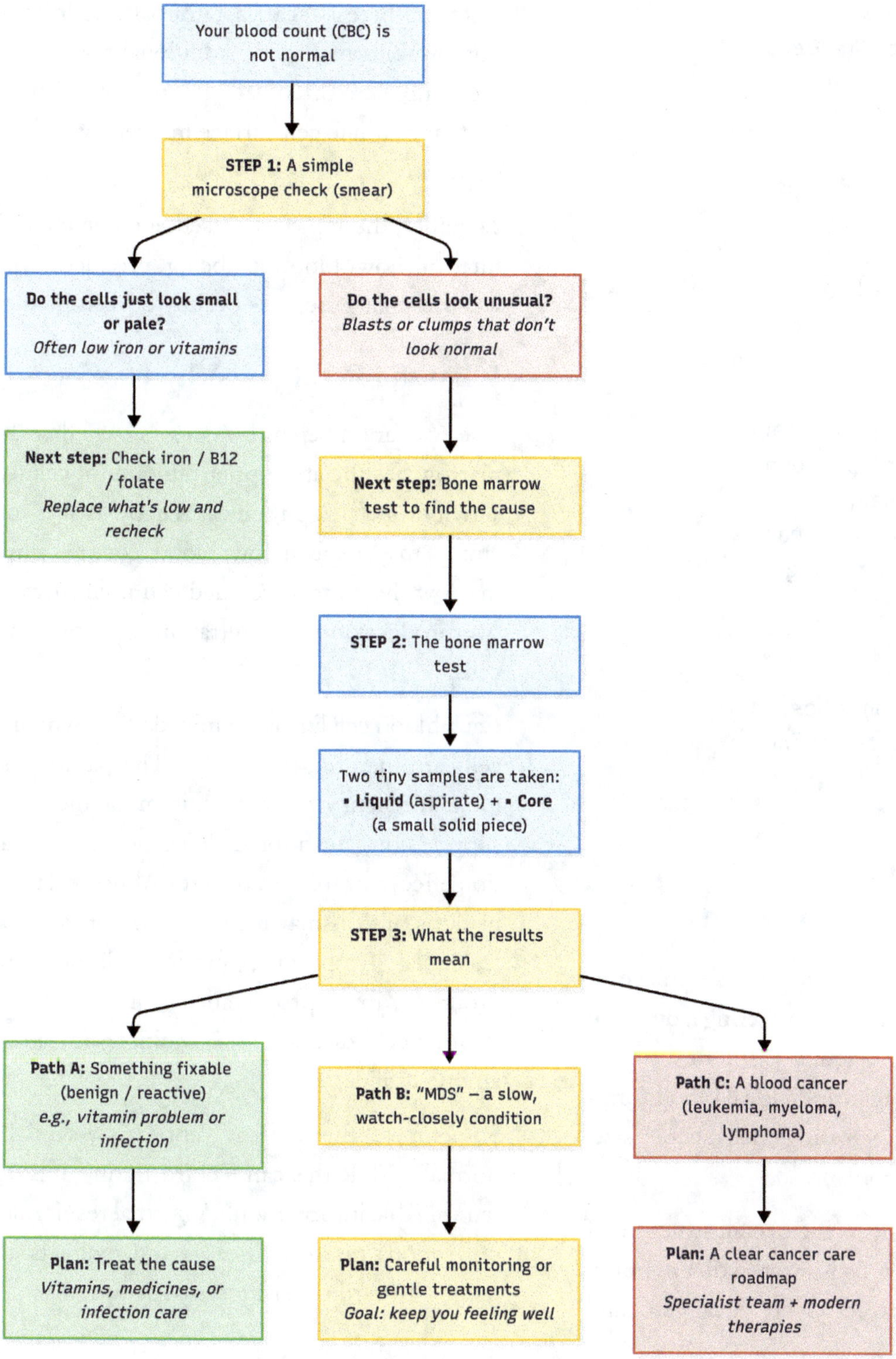
Your blood count (CBC) is not normal
STEP 1: A simple microscope check (smear)
Do the cells just look small or pale?
Often low iron or vitamins
Next step: Check iron / B12 / folate
Replace what's low and recheck
Do the cells look unusual?
Blasts or clumps that don't look normal
Next step: Bone marrow test to find the cause
STEP 2: The bone marrow test
Two tiny samples are taken:
▪ Liquid (aspirate) + ▪ Core (a small solid piece)
STEP 3: What the results mean
Path A: Something fixable (benign / reactive)
e.g., vitamin problem or infection
Plan: Treat the cause
Vitamins, medicines, or infection care
Path B: "MDS" – a slow, watch-closely condition
Plan: Careful monitoring or gentle treatments
Goal: keep you feeling well
Path C: A blood cancer (leukemia, myeloma, lymphoma)
Plan: A clear cancer care roadmap
Specialist team + modern therapies

Author Tip: The 'Deep Ache'

The Deep Bruise: Because the biopsy involves the bone itself, you may feel a 'deep ache' that is different from a skin cut.

Think of it like a significant bruise on your hip – deep, sore, and heavy. This sensation is a normal part of the bone's healing process.

It usually responds best to simple rest and avoiding pressure on that side for the night.

What Happens to the Samples

Bone marrow evaluation involves several complementary samples, each answering a different question. The liquid aspirate allows pathologists to examine individual blood forming cells in detail, assessing their shape, size, and stage of development.

The solid biopsy shows the overall structure of the marrow. It reveals how crowded the marrow space is, how cells are arranged, and whether there is scarring, fibrosis, or infiltration by abnormal cells. Additional portions of the sample are often used for specialized studies that examine cell surface markers or genetic changes.

Together, these pieces present a complete picture of how blood is being produced and whether that process is healthy or disrupted.

What the Pathologist Looks For

The evaluation begins by assessing whether the marrow has the appropriate amount of cellular activity for a person's age. Marrow that is too empty may explain low blood counts, while marrow that is too crowded can point toward overproduction or infiltration by abnormal cells.

Each blood cell line is examined to see whether cells are maturing normally. The pathologist looks for signs of infection, immune mediated suppression, nutritional deficiencies, medication effects, or toxin exposure. Abnormal populations of cells may indicate disorders such as leukemia, lymphoma, myelodysplastic syndromes, myeloproliferative disorders, or plasma cell diseases like multiple myeloma among others.

Sometimes, the marrow appears essentially normal. While this can feel frustrating, it is often valuable information. A normal result rules out serious marrow diseases and redirects attention toward other causes of symptoms.

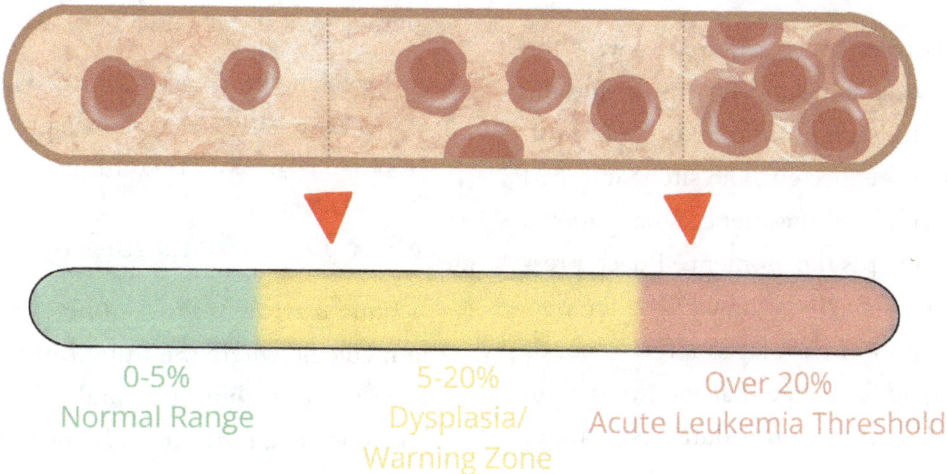

Figure 38. Illustration on how the percentage of specific cell types gives the diagnostic clue.

How Results Are Reported

Bone marrow reports can appear complex because they combine information from many tests, but the core message is usually straightforward. A report may state that the marrow is normal or reactive, meaning it is responding appropriately to stress, illness, or inflammation.

Other reports may show decreased production of one or more blood cell types, explaining low counts seen in the blood. When a specific marrow disorder or blood cancer is identified, the report names the exact diagnosis. This precision matters, because treatment decisions depend on the specific disease.

When cancer is present, the report often includes details about cell markers and genetic features that help predict how the disease is likely to behave and guide modern therapies that are increasingly targeted and effective.

What Happens Next

If the marrow is normal or shows a reversible problem, treatment may focus on correcting nutritional deficiencies, stopping or adjusting medications, or treating infections or immune conditions. In these cases, blood counts often improve once the underlying issue is addressed.

If a bone marrow disorder or blood cancer is diagnosed, the biopsy becomes the roadmap for care. Your hematologist uses the results to determine whether treatment is needed immediately, what type of therapy is most appropriate, or whether careful monitoring is the best approach.

In some situations, a repeat bone marrow biopsy is performed later. This is not because the first biopsy failed, but because marrow diseases can change over time and occasionally need reassessment.

Common Fears and Reassurances

Of all the biopsies I read, bone marrow is the one patients walk in dreading the most, and the one they often describe afterward as more tolerable than they expected. The site is numbed thoroughly with local anesthetic. What patients usually remember is the moment of deep pressure when the aspirate is drawn — a strange, sub-bone sensation that lasts a few seconds and then is over. The core that follows is similarly brief. The whole procedure takes about fifteen minutes, and most patients drive themselves home the same day.

I want to also address the fear that a diagnosis automatically means aggressive treatment, because in hematology this is often not true. Some of the chronic marrow disorders I help diagnose are monitored for years with no treatment at all. Others respond to oral medications that are now standard care. And when the marrow looks normal — which it often does, even in patients with strange blood counts — that result is not a wasted procedure. It rules out the dangerous explanations and lets the team focus on the treatable ones, like iron deficiency or recent infection, that the marrow has clearly weathered.

Example

A patient with increasing fatigue and low blood counts underwent a bone marrow biopsy. The results showed iron deficiency and a reactive marrow rather than cancer. Treating the deficiency restored normal blood counts and resolved symptoms.

In another case, repeated infections led to a biopsy that revealed acute leukemia. Because the diagnosis was made promptly, treatment began immediately and resulted in remission.

A third patient's biopsy identified multiple myeloma at an early stage, allowing timely therapy and long term disease control.

What This Means for You

A bone marrow biopsy is one of the few tests in medicine where the result can be reassuring even when nothing is found. If your marrow looks normal, it means the dangerous explanations for your abnormal counts — leukemia, lymphoma involving the marrow, infiltrative disease — have been ruled out, and your team can confidently turn to the more common and more treatable causes such as iron deficiency, vitamin B12 deficiency, medication effect, or a recent infection that the marrow has clearly weathered.

When the marrow does show a specific disorder, the path forward is more structured than most patients expect. Hematology is one of the subspecialties where the diagnosis itself dictates the treatment with unusual precision, often down to which oral medication is started or whether a watch-and-wait approach is appropriate. The discomfort of the procedure is brief; the information it returns shapes years of care. Most patients tell me afterward that the procedure was less difficult than they had feared, and that the certainty it produced was worth it.

Questions to Ask Your Doctor During a Follow-up Appointment

Understanding the Why

1. Was my marrow Hypercellular or Hypocellular? (This simply means: Is the

factory over-crowded and working too hard, or is it quiet and under-producing?)
2. Is there evidence of Fibrosis (scarring)? (Sometimes the marrow becomes fibrous, which makes it hard for new blood cells to grow.)
3. Was the finding benign (like a vitamin deficiency or infection) or malignant? (Ask if the result points to a condition like Anemia, Myelofibrosis, or a blood cancer like Leukemia or Myeloma.)
4. Is this Reactive? (Just like lymph nodes, bone marrow can work overtime reacting to a hidden infection or a medication you are taking.)

On the Result Details

1. What did the Cytogenetics show? (This is a high-tech look at the chromosomes of your marrow cells. It's often the most important part of the report for determining the exact subtype of a condition.)
2. What is the Blast Percentage? (Blasts are immature cells. A low number is normal; a high number tells the doctor the factory is sending out unfinished products.)
3. How is my Iron Store? (The biopsy can see exactly how much iron is tucked away in the marrow for future cell production.)

Next Steps

1. Do I need a Flow Cytometry report? (This is a laser-based test that identifies specific markers on the surface of your cells to give a 100% certain fingerprint of the diagnosis.)
2. Is this a condition we Watch and Wait or treat immediately? (Some marrow conditions are very slow-moving and only require a check-up every few months.)
3. Do I need to see a Hematologist-Oncologist? (These are the specialized doctors who manage factory-level blood issues.)

Recommended Bone Marrow Exam Protocol

Bone marrow health follows a Core and Liquid protocol to ensure the doctor sees both the structure of the factory and the cells it is producing.

The Peripheral Blood Trigger

- Before a marrow biopsy is ever considered, the protocol begins with a CBC (Complete Blood Count) and a Peripheral Smear.
- The Trigger: If the blood count shows blasts (baby cells) in the bloodstream, or if two or more cell lines (like red cells and platelets) are dangerously low, the protocol moves directly to a marrow biopsy.

The Aspiration and Core Protocol

A standard marrow exam almost always involves two distinct parts:

- The Aspirate (The Liquid): The doctor draws out liquid marrow. This is used for smearing on a slide to look at individual cell shapes.
- The Core (The Solid): A tiny cylinder of bone is removed. This shows the architecture, how the cells are

organized and if there is any scarring in the scaffolding of the bone.

The Blast Protocol

Pathologists use a very specific percentage to decide the next step:

- Under 5% Blasts: This is generally considered normal.
- 5% to 20% Blasts: This often triggers a protocol for Myelodysplastic Syndrome (a condition where cells don't mature correctly).
- Over 20% Blasts: This typically triggers the protocol for Acute Leukemia, requiring more urgent care.

Post-Biopsy Safety Protocol

Because the biopsy is taken from the bone, the protocol for the next 24 hours is very specific:

- Pressure at the Biopsy Site: You will have a pressure bandage applied. The protocol usually asks you to keep this bandage dry and in place for 24 hours.
- Activity: No heavy lifting or strenuous exercise for 1 to 2 days to prevent bleeding into the biopsy site.
- The Ache Expectation: It is normal to feel a deep ache in the hip (like a bad bruise) for a few days. The protocol usually suggests mild over-the-counter pain relief and rest.

Quick Summary

- Bone marrow is the body's blood factory. A biopsy is performed when blood counts are abnormal in ways that routine tests cannot explain.
- The procedure collects both a liquid (aspirate) and a solid (core) sample — together they show the marrow's individual cells and its overall structure.
- Discomfort is brief — a few seconds of deep pressure, not prolonged pain. Most patients tolerate it better than they expected.
- A normal marrow result is powerful: it rules out serious disease and lets your doctor pursue other explanations with confidence.
- When a marrow disorder is found, modern therapies are increasingly targeted; many conditions are monitored for years rather than treated aggressively.

Chapter 22

Pancreas Biopsies

Getting Answers from a Quiet Organ

What It Is and Why It's Done

The pancreas is a quiet organ. It sits deep in the abdomen, behind the stomach, and often causes no symptoms until something meaningful is happening. For this reason, pancreatic findings are often discovered on imaging done for jaundice, abdominal pain, weight loss, or even incidentally during unrelated scans.

When imaging reveals a pancreatic mass, a cyst, or an unexplained narrowing of the bile duct, a biopsy is often the only reliable way to understand what the finding truly represents. Scans can suggest possibilities, but they may not distinguish with certainty between inflammation, a benign cyst, a precancerous change, or cancer. The purpose of a pancreatic biopsy is to answer one essential question clearly and accurately: what is this? If cancer is present, identifying the exact type is critical.

How the Biopsy Is Performed

Most pancreatic biopsies are performed using endoscopic ultrasound (EUS), a technique designed specifically to reach deep organs safely. Biopsy can also be done during an endoscopic retrograde cholangio-pancreaticography (ERCP).

While you are comfortably sedated, a gastroenterologist passes a flexible scope through the mouth into the stomach or small intestine. An ultrasound probe at the tip of the scope allows the pancreas to be seen clearly through the wall of the digestive tract.

Using this real time imaging, the doctor guides a very thin needle directly into the area of concern and collects cells or small tissue fragments. This approach avoids skin incisions and keeps the procedure minimally invasive. In selected cases, particularly when EUS is not feasible, a CT guided needle biopsy through the skin may be used instead. After the procedure, patients are monitored briefly and typically go home the same day.

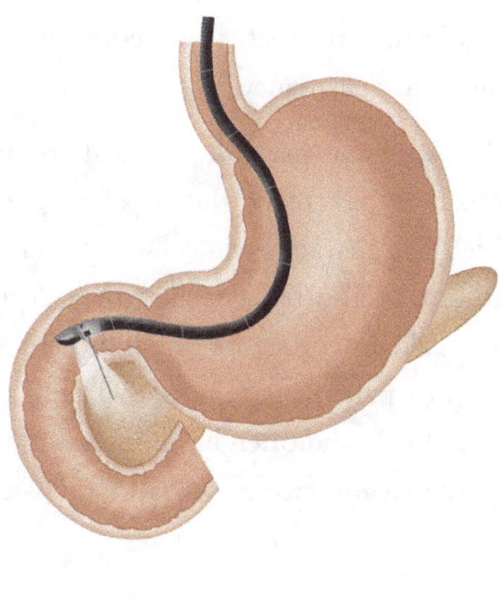

Figure 39. Endoscopic ultrasound guided biopsy of pancreatic tumor.

In the Pathology Laboratory

Pancreatic biopsies are usually FNA aspirates — clouds of individual cells rather than coherent tissue cores. The cells are carefully spread onto glass slides so the pathologist can examine them in detail. When possible, additional material is collected to prepare a cell block, which allows further testing to be performed.

Because pancreatic samples are often small and the lesions themselves can be subtle, careful handling is essential. Just as important is correlation with imaging findings. The pathologist works closely with the procedural and imaging teams to ensure that the microscopic findings match what was seen on scans.

What the Pathologist Looks For

The first task is to determine whether the sample represents benign inflammation, reactive change, or a true tumor. This distinction can be challenging. Conditions such as chronic pancreatitis, an inflammation, can distort cells and mimic cancer, so the pathologist looks for specific features that separate injury and scarring from malignancy.

When cancer is present, the most common diagnosis is pancreatic ductal adenocarcinoma, which has characteristic cellular patterns. The pathologist also remains alert for a type of tumors called neuroendocrine tumors; a distinct group of pancreatic tumors that tend to grow more slowly and often have different, more favorable treatment options. In biopsies from cystic lesions, the cells are evaluated to determine whether the cyst is harmless or carries potential for becoming cancerous.

How Results Are Reported

Like every other report, pancreatic biopsy reports are written to be direct and clinically useful. A result may be negative for malignancy, often due to inflammation or a benign cyst. Sometimes the result is described as atypical or suspicious, indicating that the cells are abnormal but limited in number; in these cases, repeat sampling or close follow up is often recommended.

A malignant result confirms cancer and names the type, such as pancreatic ductal adenocarcinoma or neuroendocrine tumor. When possible, the report also comments on whether the biopsy findings explain what was seen on imaging, a crucial step in determining whether the sample is representative.

What Happens Next

If the biopsy is benign, your care team may recommend monitoring with imaging or treatment of underlying inflammation. When results are uncertain, additional imaging or repeat biopsy may be advised, particularly if clinical suspicion remains high.

When cancer is diagnosed, the biopsy becomes the foundation for everything that follows. It determines whether surgery is an option, which medications are most likely to help, and whether additional testing is needed to personalize treatment. In this way, the biopsy guides both the urgency and the direction of care.

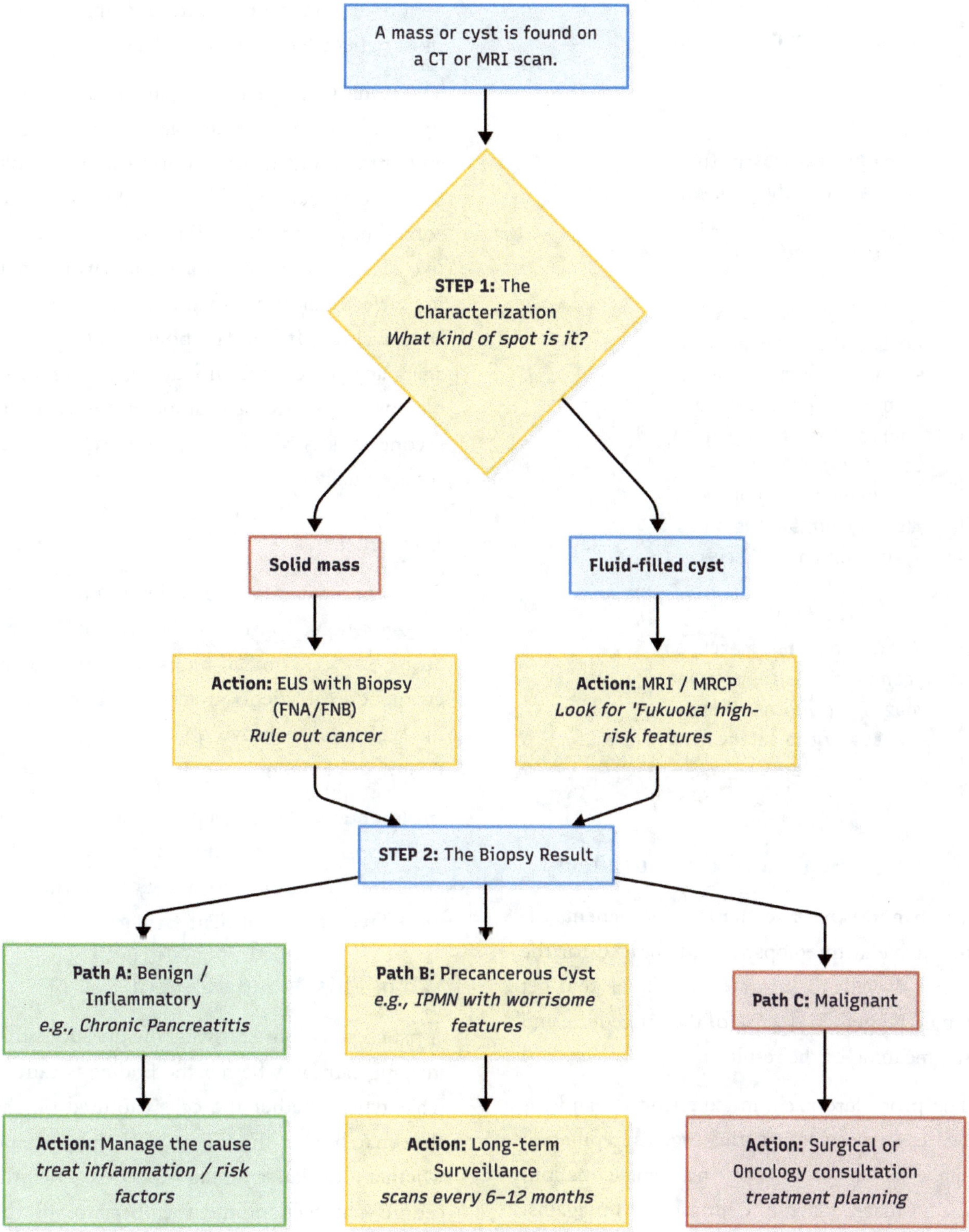
A mass or cyst is found on a CT or MRI scan.
STEP 1: The Characterization
What kind of spot is it?
Solid mass
Fluid-filled cyst
Action: EUS with Biopsy (FNA/FNB)
Rule out cancer
Action: MRI / MRCP
Look for 'Fukuoka' high-risk features
STEP 2: The Biopsy Result
Path A: Benign / Inflammatory
e.g., Chronic Pancreatitis
Path B: Precancerous Cyst
e.g., IPMN with worrisome features
Path C: Malignant
Action: Manage the cause
treat inflammation / risk factors
Action: Long-term Surveillance
scans every 6–12 months
Action: Surgical or Oncology consultation
treatment planning

> **Author Tip: Correlation is Key**
>
> **The Perfect Match:** In pancreatic pathology, we always ask: *'Does the slide match the scan?'*
>
> Because these samples are so small, one of the most important parts of your report is the doctor's note confirming that the cells found on the biopsy actually explain the mass seen on your CT scan.
>
> If the two do **not** match, a second look – either repeat imaging or another biopsy – is usually the safest next step.

Common Fears and Reassurances

The pancreas has a reputation, and patients often arrive at the biopsy already braced for the worst. I want to separate two things that get tangled together: the risk of the procedure, and the meaning of the result.

The procedure itself, in experienced hands, is far less invasive than the organ's reputation suggests. The endoscopist passes a scope into the stomach, places the ultrasound tip against the stomach wall directly opposite the pancreas, and threads a thin needle through that wall into the lesion. There is no skin incision and no path through the abdominal cavity. Serious complications are uncommon, and most patients go home the same day.

The result is where I want patients to keep an open mind. The pancreas is a fibrotic organ, and chronic inflammation in it can look strikingly like cancer on a CT scan, on an MRI, and sometimes on the first biopsy as well. A negative result in the face of a suspicious image is not a clean bill of health and not a wasted procedure either. It is a data point. When the imaging and the cells do not agree, the responsible answer is often to sample again, and that second look is where many pancreatic diagnoses are finally made.

Example

A patient developed unexplained jaundice, and imaging showed a mass in the head of the pancreas. An EUS guided biopsy confirmed pancreatic ductal adenocarcinoma, allowing the medical team to move quickly to staging and treatment planning.

In another patient, a small pancreatic lesion was biopsied and diagnosed as a neuroendocrine tumor, leading to a very different, and more favorable, treatment strategy.

What This Means for You

A pancreatic biopsy answers the questions that imaging cannot: whether the finding is cancer, what type, whether the cells captured on the slide match what the CT or MRI showed, and whether a repeat sampling is needed. The procedure can feel intimidating because of the pancreas's reputation, but the modern endoscopic approach is well-tolerated, and the slides that result are what shift the conversation from speculation to oncology planning.

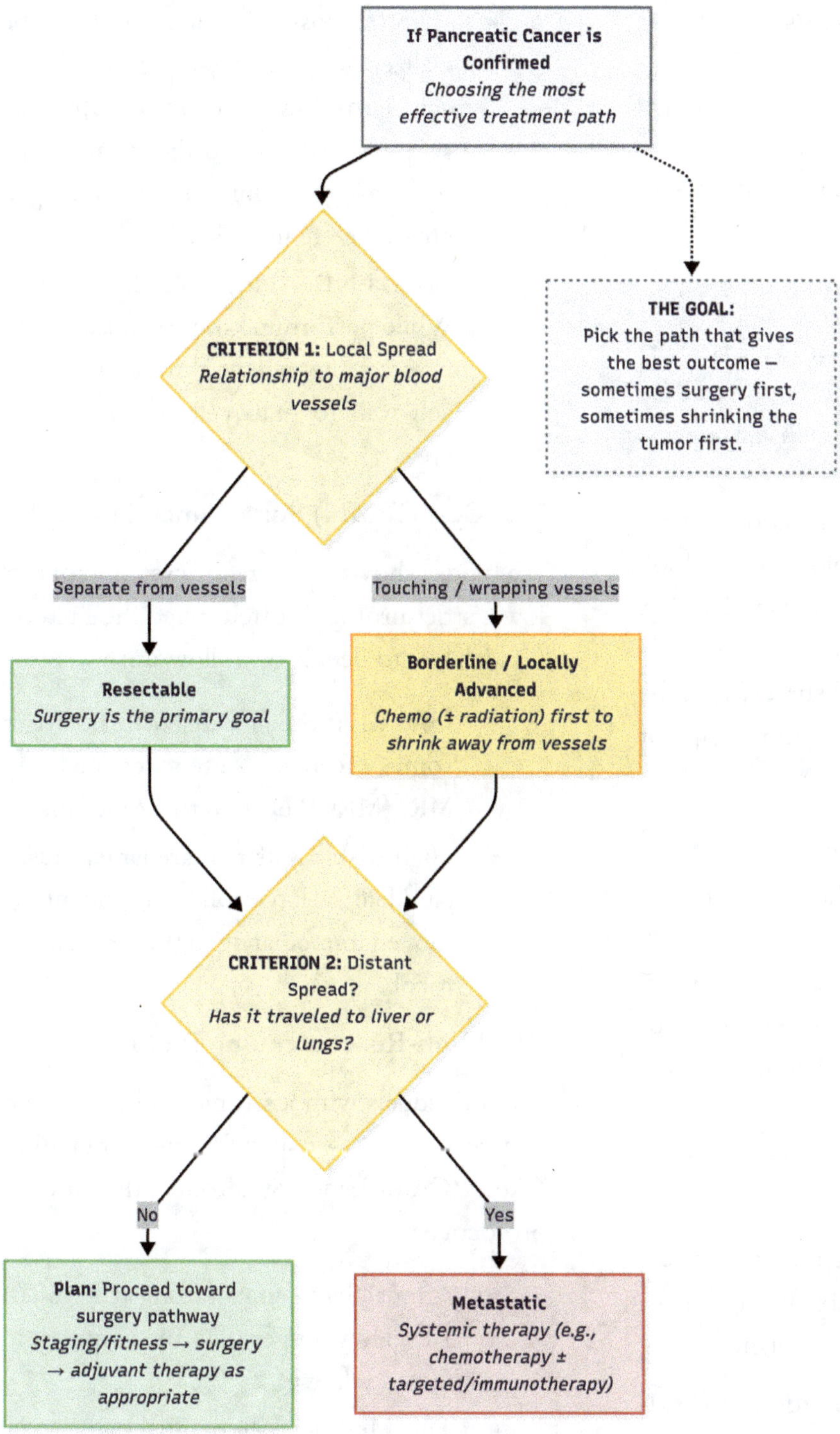

Questions to Ask Your Doctor During a Follow-up Appointment

Understanding the Pathology

1. What was the specific diagnosis? (e.g., Is it Adenocarcinoma, a Neuroendocrine Tumor (NET), or a benign cyst?)
2. If it is a cyst, what type is it? (Some cysts, like IPMNs, have a small risk of turning into cancer, while others, like

serous cystadenomas, are almost always harmless.)
3. Was the sample sufficient? (Pancreatic samples can be tiny; ask if there was enough tissue to run all necessary tests.)

On Treatment and Next Steps

1. Is the growth resectable? (This is a surgical term asking if the spot can be completely removed with an operation.)
2. Do I need additional blood work? (Sometimes we use a blood test to look for pancreatic cancer markers like CA 19-9 to support the tissue results.)
3. What are the options if surgery isn't the first step? (Ask about chemotherapy or radiation before surgery.)

Long-Term Monitoring

1. If it's a low-risk cyst, how often do we need to scan it?
2. Should I have genetic testing? (Certain pancreatic findings are linked to hereditary markers like BRCA mutations.)

Recommended Pancreatic Exam Protocol

Because the pancreas is deep in the body, health protocols rely on a combination of high-tech imaging and risk-based surveillance.

The First-Look Protocol (Incidental Findings)

Most pancreatic issues are found incidentally when a patient gets a CT scan for an unrelated reason (like back pain or a kidney stone). The protocol then triggers:

- EUS (Endoscopic Ultrasound): A specialized scope is passed into the stomach. An ultrasound on the tip of the scope looks through the stomach wall to get a high-definition view of the pancreas. See figure 39 above.
- FNA/FNB (Fine Needle Biopsy): While performing the EUS, the doctor passes a tiny needle through the stomach wall to grab cells from the pancreas.

The Cyst (IPMN) Surveillance Protocol

If a biopsy shows a pancreatic cyst, doctors follow a strict protocol (often called the Fukuoka Guidelines) to decide on follow-up:

- Low Risk: Small cysts with no worrisome features are scanned via MRI/MRCP every 6 to 12 months.
- High Risk: Cysts that are large, causing jaundice, or have solid components are moved immediately to the surgical protocol.

The High-Risk Screening Protocol

For individuals with a strong family history of pancreatic cancer or specific genetic mutations (like BRCA or Lynch Syndrome), the universal protocol is:

- Annual Screening: Starting at age 50 (or 10 years younger than the youngest affected relative).
- The Method: Alternating between an MRI/MRCP and an Endoscopic Ultrasound (EUS) every year.

Post-Biopsy Safety Protocol

The pancreas is a sensitive organ that produces digestive enzymes. The primary concern after a biopsy is pancreatitis (temporary inflammation). The protocol includes:

- Enzyme Monitoring: Occasionally checking for abdominal pain or nausea.
- Observation: Staying in the recovery area for a few hours to ensure you can drink fluids and have no significant pain.
- Activity: Avoiding heavy meals and strenuous activity for the first 24 to 48 hours.

Quick Summary

- The pancreas sits deep in the abdomen and rarely causes symptoms early. Most masses are found incidentally on imaging or after jaundice appears.
- Most pancreatic biopsies are done via endoscopic ultrasound (EUS) — a scope passes into the stomach so a needle can reach the pancreas through the stomach wall, with no skin incision.
- The biopsy distinguishes chronic inflammation (which can mimic cancer) from adenocarcinoma (the most common pancreatic cancer) and neuroendocrine tumors (slower-growing, very different treatment).
- Pancreatic cysts are managed using established surveillance guidelines based on size and worrisome features — most are watched with periodic MRI rather than removed.
- A negative biopsy in the face of suspicious imaging does not mean the finding is dismissed; repeat sampling is a normal and responsible next step.

Chapter 23

Vulvar Biopsies

Sorting Chronic Symptoms from Serious Disease

What It Is and Why It's Done

The vulva is exposed to moisture, friction, inflammation, hormonal shifts, and age-related skin changes. Because of this, symptoms such as itching, burning, color changes, thickening of the skin, or sores are common and, in many cases, caused by benign conditions.

At the same time, some vulvar disorders represent precancerous or cancerous changes that benefit from early identification. These conditions can look very similar to non-cancerous inflammation on visual examination alone. Vulvar biopsies are performed when symptoms persist despite treatment, worsen over time, or when a visible lesion raises concern.

The biopsy provides a clear distinction between inflammatory conditions, precancerous changes, and cancer. Rather than relying solely on appearance or symptoms, it allows direct examination of the tissue so that serious disease is not missed and benign conditions are treated appropriately.

How the Biopsy Is Performed

A vulvar biopsy is a targeted and usually brief procedure. After the area is numbed with a local anesthetic, a small piece of tissue is removed from the area of concern. Because the vulva is visible and accessible, the biopsy can be selected with precision.

Mild soreness is common afterward, particularly for the first day or two, but discomfort is generally short lived. Healing typically occurs within days, and most patients return quickly to normal activities with simple care instructions.

In the Pathology Laboratory

Once the biopsy reaches the pathology laboratory, it is carefully processed so that both the surface skin and the deeper supporting tissue can be examined. This depth assessment is important for all vulvar biopsies, but it is especially critical when cancer is a concern.

If invasive cancer is identified, the depth of invasion is measured in millimeters. This single measurement plays a major role in determining treatment, surgical planning, and prognosis. Careful processing ensures that this depth can be assessed accurately and reliably.

What the Pathologist Looks For

Many vulvar biopsies show benign inflammatory skin conditions. One common example is lichen sclerosus, a chronic inflammatory condition that can cause intense itching, skin thinning, and architectural changes but is not itself cancerous. While symptoms can be severe, proper diagnosis allows effective treatment and long term management.

The pathologist also evaluates for vulvar intraepithelial neoplasia, often abbreviated as VIN. VIN represents a precancerous change in which abnormal cells are confined to the surface layers of the skin. VIN is graded as VIN-I, II, or III depending on the severity of the dysplasia. This allows treatment before invasion occurs.

If abnormal cells have breached normal tissue boundaries and extend into deeper tissue, the diagnosis is invasive squamous cell carcinoma, the most common vulvar cancer. The distinction between surface limited disease and invasive cancer is central to determining the next steps in care.

How Results Are Reported

Your report will name the diagnosis directly and describe what it means clinically. Common results include inflammatory skin disorders, precancerous changes, and invasive cancer.

When cancer is present, additional details are included, most importantly the depth of invasion and whether abnormal cells extend to the edges of the biopsy. These measurements guide treatment decisions and help determine whether further procedures are needed.

Each reported element is chosen because it influences care, not simply because it can be described.

What Happens Next

When inflammatory conditions are diagnosed, treatment focuses on symptom relief and long term control, often with topical medications and careful follow up. Appropriate therapy can significantly improve quality of life and reduce ongoing irritation.

When precancerous lesions are identified, treatment is recommended to prevent progression. These treatments are typically localized and effective.

If vulvar cancer is detected early, treatment can often be limited and highly successful. Early diagnosis frequently allows smaller procedures, better healing, and excellent long-term outcomes.

Common Fears and Reassurances

The vulvar biopsies that come to my desk often arrive after years of symptoms — itching, burning, a patch of skin that has changed over time and never quite settled. Patients have usually tried over-the-counter creams, sometimes prescription ones, and have lived with the discomfort longer than they should have, often because they were afraid of what a biopsy might find. I understand the avoidance. The location is private, and the worry tends to grow in silence.

What I want to say plainly is that most of the vulvar biopsies I read are not cancer. The majority describe lichen sclerosus, an inflammatory skin condition that responds well to high-potency topical steroids once correctly identified. Others show different reactive or inflammatory patterns that have explanations and treatments. A small fraction show vulvar intraepithelial neoplasia, a true precancer that can be treated locally. The biopsy is a small, well-tolerated procedure done under local anesthesia. The years of guessing it ends are often a bigger relief than patients expected.

Example

A patient with longstanding vulvar itching underwent biopsy after symptoms failed to improve with initial treatment. The biopsy showed lichen sclerosus rather than cancer. With appropriate therapy, symptoms improved significantly, and the patient entered a plan for ongoing monitoring to watch for future changes.

What This Means for You

Vulvar biopsies turn persistent symptoms into clear answers. Whether a condition is inflammatory, precancerous, or cancerous, identifying it early allows care to be focused, effective, and timely.

Instead of continued guessing or untreated discomfort, the biopsy provides direction. It supports appropriate treatment, reduces unnecessary worry, and protects long term health through precise diagnosis and thoughtful follow up.

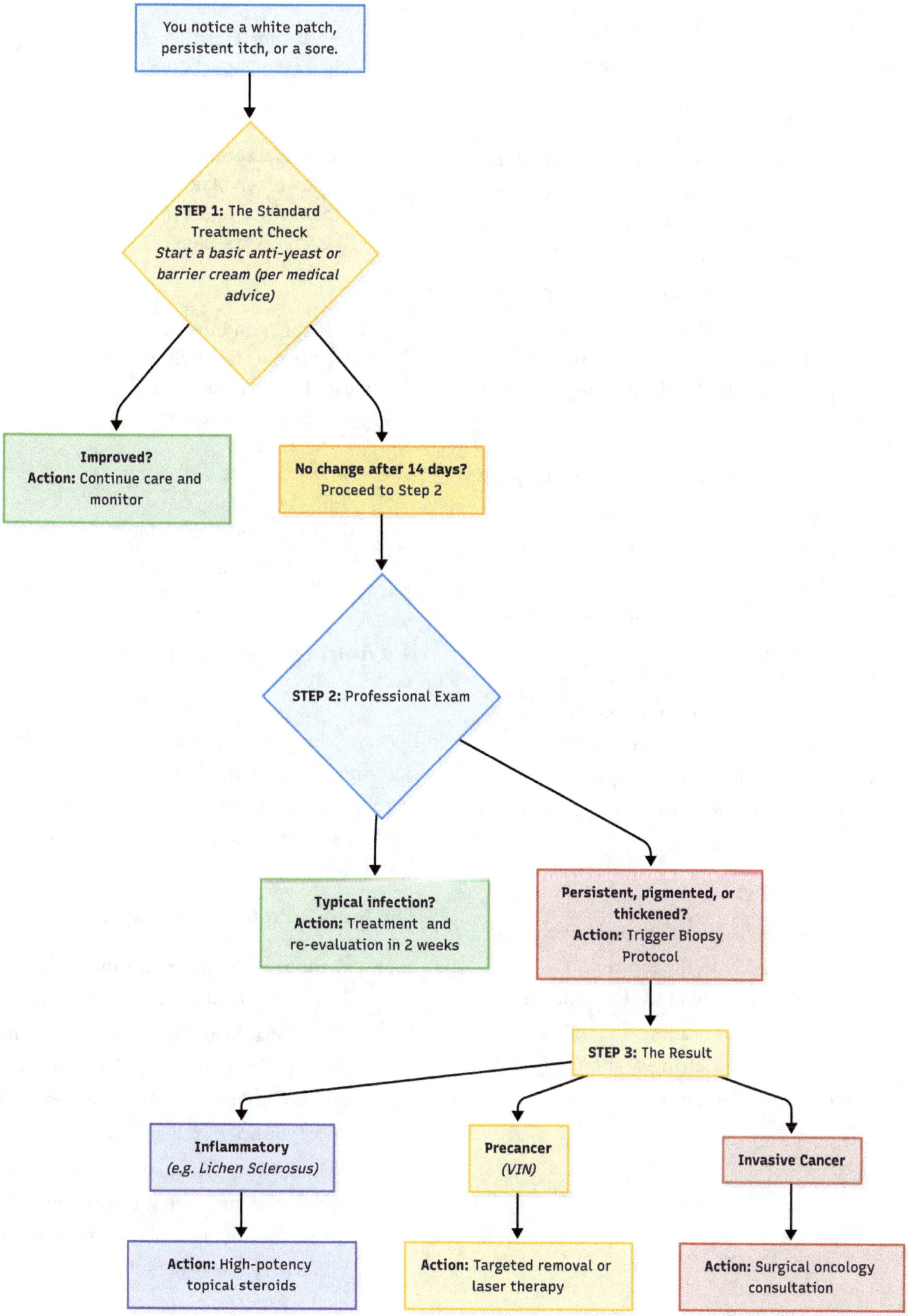
You notice a white patch, persistent itch, or a sore.
STEP 1: The Standard Treatment Check
Start a basic anti-yeast or barrier cream (per medical advice)
Improved?
Action: Continue care and monitor
No change after 14 days?
Proceed to Step 2
STEP 2: Professional Exam
Typical infection?
Action: Treatment and re-evaluation in 2 weeks
Persistent, pigmented, or thickened?
Action: Trigger Biopsy Protocol
STEP 3: The Result
Inflammatory
(e.g. Lichen Sclerosus)
Precancer
(VIN)
Invasive Cancer
Action: High-potency topical steroids
Action: Targeted removal or laser therapy
Action: Surgical oncology consultation

Questions to Ask Your Doctor During a Follow-up Appointment

Understanding the Results

1. What is the name of the condition found? (Common results include Lichen Sclerosus, Lichen Planus, or Vulvar Intraepithelial Neoplasia (VIN).)
2. Is this an inflammatory condition or a precancerous change?
3. Is the condition localized to the biopsy spot, or is it likely affecting bigger area?

Treatment and Management

1. What is the best way to treat this? (For example, many vulvar conditions respond well to high-potency steroid ointments.)
2. Is this a chronic condition I will need to manage long-term?
3. How do I apply medications to such a sensitive area? (Ask for specific instructions on quantity and frequency.)
4. Are there lifestyle changes, like using different soaps or wearing specific fabrics, that will help?

Future Monitoring

1. Does this diagnosis increase my risk for vulvar cancer in the future?
2. How often should I have a professional vulvar map or exam?
3. What specific changes should I look for during a self-exam at home?

> 💡 **Author Tip: The 'Cigarette Paper' Clue**
>
> **Texture Matters:** Lichen Sclerosus often makes the skin look white and shiny – like 'cigarette paper.'
>
> If the skin looks translucent, fragile, or unusually thin, don't wait for it to become painful.
>
> **Early treatment** can prevent long-term scarring or the skin fusing together.

Recommended Vulvar Exam Protocol

Because the vulva is technically specialized skin, the protocol combines elements of dermatology and gynecology. Doctors follow a Look, Feel, and Sample protocol to ensure health.

The Annual Professional Inspection

- A thorough vulvar exam should be part of every annual gynecological visit.
- The Visual Map: The clinician looks for changes in symmetry, skin thickness, and color (such as white patches, dark spots, or bright red areas).
- Magnification: If a spot is suspicious, the doctor may use a colposcope (the same magnifying tool used for the cervix) to get a high-definition view of the skin's surface.

The Monthly Mirror Self-Exam

Dermatologists recommend checking your moles; gynecologists recommend checking the vulva. Once a month, use a hand mirror in a well-lit room to check for:

- The Two-Week Rule: Any sore, ulcer, or cut that does not heal within 14 days needs a professional evaluation.
- The Itch That Won't Quit: Persistent itching that doesn't respond to over-the-counter yeast infection treatments is a primary trigger for a biopsy.
- Color Changes: Specifically, look for patches that are much whiter, darker, or thicker than the surrounding skin.

The Biopsy Trigger: The Rule of Persistent Change

The universal protocol dictates that a biopsy should be performed if:

- A lesion does not respond to initial standard treatment (like a basic anti-fungal or mild steroid).
- A spot is pigmented (darker than the rest) and has irregular borders.
- The skin appears cigarette-paper thin or has become fused or scarred.

VIN Management

If a biopsy shows VIN, the protocol shifts to active management:

- Grading: Similar to the cervix, VIN is graded 1, 2, or 3.
- Treatment: Higher grades (2 and 3) are typically treated with surgical removal, laser therapy, or specialized topical creams to prevent progression to cancer.
- Frequency: Follow-up exams usually occur every 3 to 6 months for the first few years after treatment.

Quick Summary

- Many vulvar symptoms — itching, white patches, soreness — come from benign inflammatory conditions like lichen sclerosus rather than cancer.
- Biopsy is the only reliable way to tell benign inflammation, precancerous changes (VIN), and early cancer apart; they look very similar to the eye.
- If cancer is found, the depth of invasion in millimeters is the single most important number — it determines surgical planning more than tumor size.
- Most chronic vulvar conditions respond well to targeted treatments (often topical steroids) once correctly diagnosed.
- Any sore or unhealed area lasting more than two weeks, or persistent itching that doesn't respond to standard treatment, warrants professional evaluation.

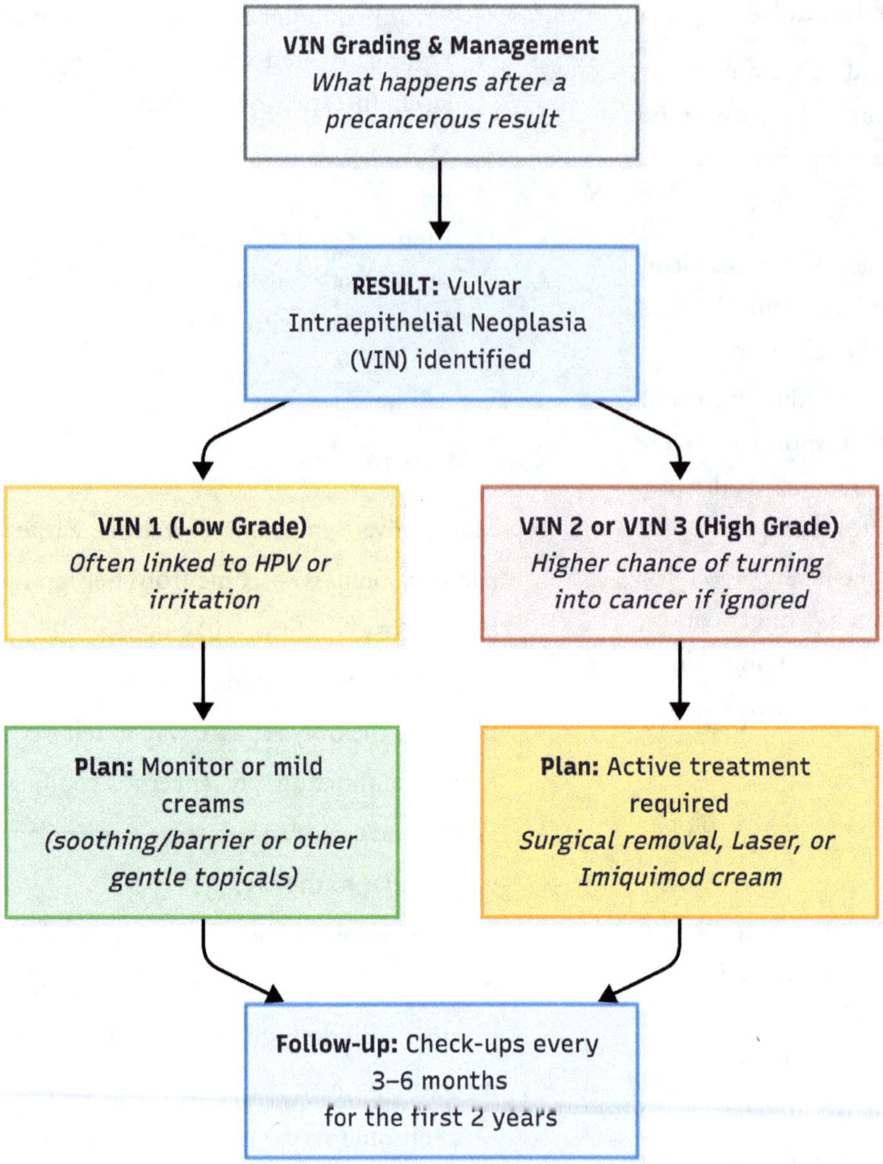

VIN Grading & Management
What happens after a precancerous result
RESULT: Vulvar Intraepithelial Neoplasia (VIN) identified
VIN 1 (Low Grade)
Often linked to HPV or irritation
VIN 2 or VIN 3 (High Grade)
Higher chance of turning into cancer if ignored
Plan: Monitor or mild creams
(soothing/barrier or other gentle topicals)
Plan: Active treatment required
Surgical removal, Laser, or Imiquimod cream
Follow-Up: Check-ups every 3–6 months for the first 2 years

Chapter 24

Penile Biopsies

Sorting Persistent Changes from Serious Disease

What It Is and Why It's Done

The skin of the penis is unique, highly specialized, and sensitive. Like the rest of the body's protective barrier, it is exposed to friction, moisture, and potential irritants; however, it is also subject to specific hormonal environments and viral exposures. Because of this, it is common to experience symptoms such as persistent itching, redness, white patches, or small sores. In many cases, these issues are caused by benign inflammatory conditions or common infections.

At the same time, certain penile disorders represent precancerous changes or early-stage cancer. On visual examination alone, a harmless inflammatory patch can look remarkably similar to a high-risk lesion. A penile biopsy is performed when a spot does not heal with standard creams, when a lesion changes color or texture, or when an unexplained growth appears.

The biopsy provides the definitive distinction between a chronic skin condition and a malignancy. Biopsy allows a pathologist to look at the tissue architecture directly, ensuring that serious disease is caught early and that benign conditions are managed with the correct medications.

How the Biopsy Is Performed

A penile biopsy is a targeted, outpatient procedure that usually takes less than fifteen minutes. Because the area is highly sensitive, the clinician first applies a numbing cream or injects a local anesthetic to ensure the patient is comfortable. Once the area is numb, a small punch or shave of tissue is removed from the most suspicious part of the lesion.

Because the penis is easily accessible, the biopsy can be selected with extreme precision. In some cases, a small stitch may be required to close the site, while in others, the area is allowed to heal on its own like a small scrape. Mild soreness or bruising is common for a few days, but most patients return to their normal routine quickly with simple care instructions, such as keeping the area clean and dry.

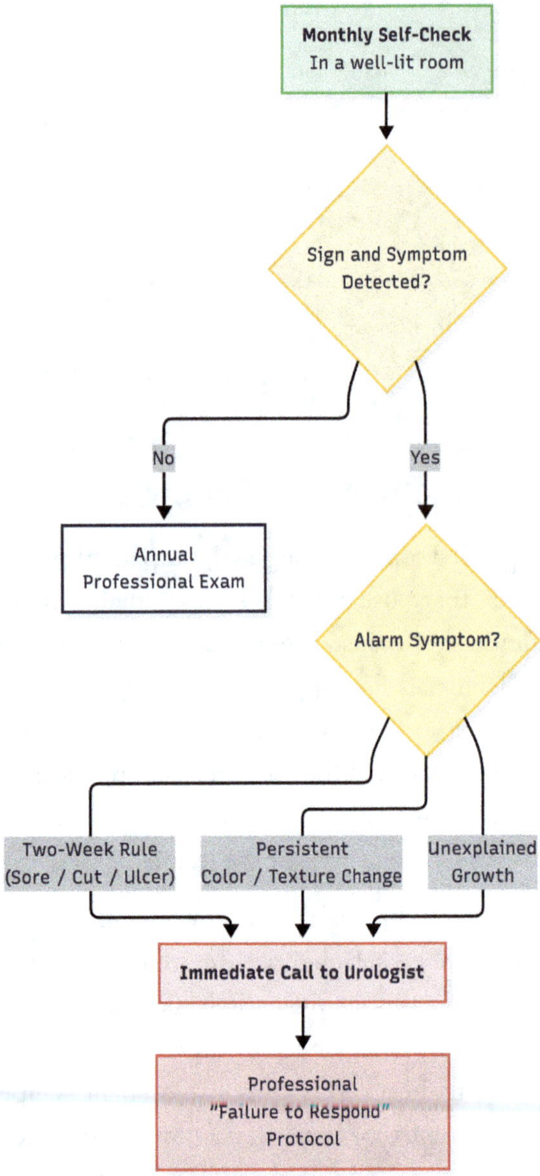

In the Pathology Laboratory

When the sample reaches the lab, it is processed so that the pathologist can see the full stack of tissue. This includes the topmost surface (the epithelium) and the deeper supporting layers (the dermis). This vertical view is essential.

The pathologist must determine if abnormal cells are staying strictly on the surface or if they have begun to root into the deeper tissue. If invasive cancer is identified, the depth of invasion is measured in millimeters. Much like a property line, this measurement is the single most important factor in deciding whether the patient needs simple local treatment or a more extensive surgical approach.

What the Pathologist Looks For

Many penile biopsies reveal benign, though frustrating, inflammatory conditions. One frequent diagnosis is lichen sclerosus (sometimes called balanitis xerotica obliterans or BXO). This is a chronic inflammatory condition that causes white, thinned-out patches and scarring. While it is not cancer, it can cause significant discomfort and, if left untreated, can increase the risk of future cellular changes.

The pathologist also looks for Penile Intraepithelial Neoplasia (PeIN), the penile counterpart of VIN. This is a precancerous state where abnormal, disorganized cells are found within the skin's surface but have not yet breached the deeper layers. Identifying PeIN is a win for the patient, as it allows for highly effective treatment before a true cancer can form.

If the abnormal cells have moved past the surface barrier, the diagnosis becomes Invasive Squamous Cell Carcinoma. By examining the shape and growth pattern of these cells, the pathologist can grade the cancer, telling the medical team how aggressively the cells are behaving.

How Results Are Reported

Penile pathology reports are designed to be a roadmap for the urologist. The report will state the diagnosis clearly, but it also includes margin information. If the abnormal cells go right to the edge of the biopsy sample, it suggests the lesion may be larger than what was sampled.

For cancer cases, the report will specify the Subtype. Some versions of penile cancer are linked to the Human Papillomavirus (HPV), while others are not. Knowing the subtype helps the doctor predict how the condition will respond to different therapies, such as specialized creams, laser treatment, or surgery.

What Happens Next

If the result is inflammatory (like Lichen Sclerosus): Treatment focuses on high-potency topical steroids to calm the immune response and prevent scarring. Regular follow-ups are scheduled to ensure the skin remains healthy.

If the result is precancerous (PeIN): The doctor may use organ-sparing treatments. This can include medicated creams that trigger the immune system to destroy the bad cells, or precise laser therapy.

If the result is invasive cancer: The biopsy results dictate the surgical plan. Because of modern pathology, many patients can undergo limited procedures that remove only the diseased tissue while preserving as much healthy function and appearance as possible.

Common Fears Patients Have

Penile biopsies are the cases where the patient has most often waited the longest before walking through the door. The location, the embarrassment, the fear of what the doctor might find and what the doctor might do — all of it conspires to keep men quiet about a patch or a lesion that has been changing for months or years. I want to address that quietness directly, because waiting is the only thing about this category of disease that makes the outcomes worse.

The biopsy itself is small. A punch or a shave under local anesthetic, a stitch sometimes, an outpatient procedure. What it returns is information that almost always works in the patient's favor. Most lesions I read are inflammatory conditions like lichen sclerosus, which respond to topical steroids. Some are precancerous changes — penile intraepithelial neoplasia — which are typically treated with creams or limited local procedures that preserve the organ entirely. The radical surgeries men fear are the destination of late disease, not the destination of a biopsy. The biopsy is the off-ramp.

Example

A patient noticed a persistent red patch that didn't go away with over-the-counter anti-fungal cream. After a visit with a urologist, a small punch biopsy was performed, which identified Penile Intraepithelial Neoplasia (PeIN) (a precancerous lesion). Because it was caught before it became invasive cancer, he was treated with a specialized topical cream for several weeks. Follow-up biopsies showed the area was clear, and he avoided surgery entirely.

What This Means for You

A penile biopsy turns a spot of concern into a plan of action. Whether the result is a manageable skin condition or a more serious change, the biopsy provides the clarity needed to choose the most effective, least invasive path forward. What it replaces, more often than not, is years of avoidance — with a treatment plan small enough to fit on a tube of cream.

Questions to Ask Your Doctor During a Follow-up Appointment

Understanding the Results

1. What is the specific name of the condition identified? (Common results may include Lichen Sclerosus, Penile Intraepithelial Neoplasia (PeIN), or Squamous Cell Carcinoma.)
2. If the pathology showed cancer, was the finding In-Situ or Invasive? (This distinguishes if abnormal cells are strictly on the surface or have moved into deeper tissue.)
3. If PeIN, what was the Grade of the cells? (The pathologist assigns a grade of 1, 2, or 3 to show how aggressively the cells are going upwards to the surface compared to normal skin.)
4. Does the report mention Margins? (This confirms if the entire abnormal area was captured or if the lesion likely extends beyond the biopsy site.)
5. Is this condition related to a previous viral infection, such as HPV? (Knowing the subtype helps determine the most effective therapy.)

Treatment and Management

1. Is an organ-sparing approach an option for me? (Ask if the condition can be treated with specialized creams, laser ablation, or Mohs surgery rather than more extensive procedures.)
2. How should I apply topical medications to such a sensitive area? (Request specific instructions on the frequency and the exact amount of ointment to use.)
3. If this is an inflammatory condition like Lichen Sclerosus, is it chronic? (Understand if you will need long-term management with steroids to prevent scarring.)
4. Are there specific irritants I should avoid? (Ask if changes in soaps, detergents, or lubricants are necessary to aid healing.)

Future Monitoring

1. Does this diagnosis increase my long-term risk for penile cancer?
2. How often do I need a professional skin map or follow-up exam? (Standard surveillance often occurs every 3 to 6 months for the first two years after a PeIN or cancer diagnosis.)
3. What specific changes should I look for during my monthly self-exams?
4. When does the Two-Week Rule apply to me? (Confirm if any new sore or color change that doesn't heal within 14 days should trigger an immediate call.)

Recommended Penile Exam Protocol

Urologists and dermatologists follow a specific Look, Feel, and Sample protocol to maintain penile health.

The Monthly Self-Check

Just as men are encouraged to perform testicular self-exams, a monthly skin check is vital. In a well-lit room, look for:

- The Two-Week Rule: Any sore, cut, or ulcer that does not heal within 14 days requires professional evaluation.
- Texture Changes: Patches that feel much harder, thicker, or velvety compared to the surrounding skin.
- Color Shifts: New white, bright red, or dark brown/black spots.

The Biopsy Trigger

The universal protocol dictates a biopsy must be performed if:

- A lesion does not resolve after a 2-to-4-week course of standard treatment (like a basic steroid or anti-fungal cream).
- A spot appears wart-like but does not respond to typical wart treatments.
- The skin appears scarred or causes a tightening that interferes with normal function.

PeIN / Cancer Management Protocol

If the biopsy shows precancerous or cancerous changes, the protocol shifts to staging and precision care:

- Grading: The pathologist assigns a grade (1, 2, or 3) to show how much the cells look like normal skin.
- Organ-Sparing Approach: Whenever possible, the protocol favors treatments that preserve tissue, such as Mohs surgery, laser ablation, or topical chemotherapy.
- Surveillance: After treatment, follow-up exams occur every 3 to 6 months for the first two years to catch any recurrence at the earliest possible moment.

Quick Summary

- A penile biopsy prevents radical surgery rather than causing it — finding precancer (PeIN) early allows treatment with creams or laser rather than larger procedures.
- Many lesions are benign inflammatory conditions (like lichen sclerosus / BXO) that respond well to topical steroids once correctly diagnosed.
- The depth of invasion is the key measurement that determines whether local treatment is sufficient or more extensive surgery is needed.
- Modern care strongly favors organ-sparing approaches — creams, laser, Mohs surgery — whenever the diagnosis allows it.
- Any sore, ulcer, or new patch that does not heal within two weeks, or fails to respond to standard creams within a month, needs professional evaluation.

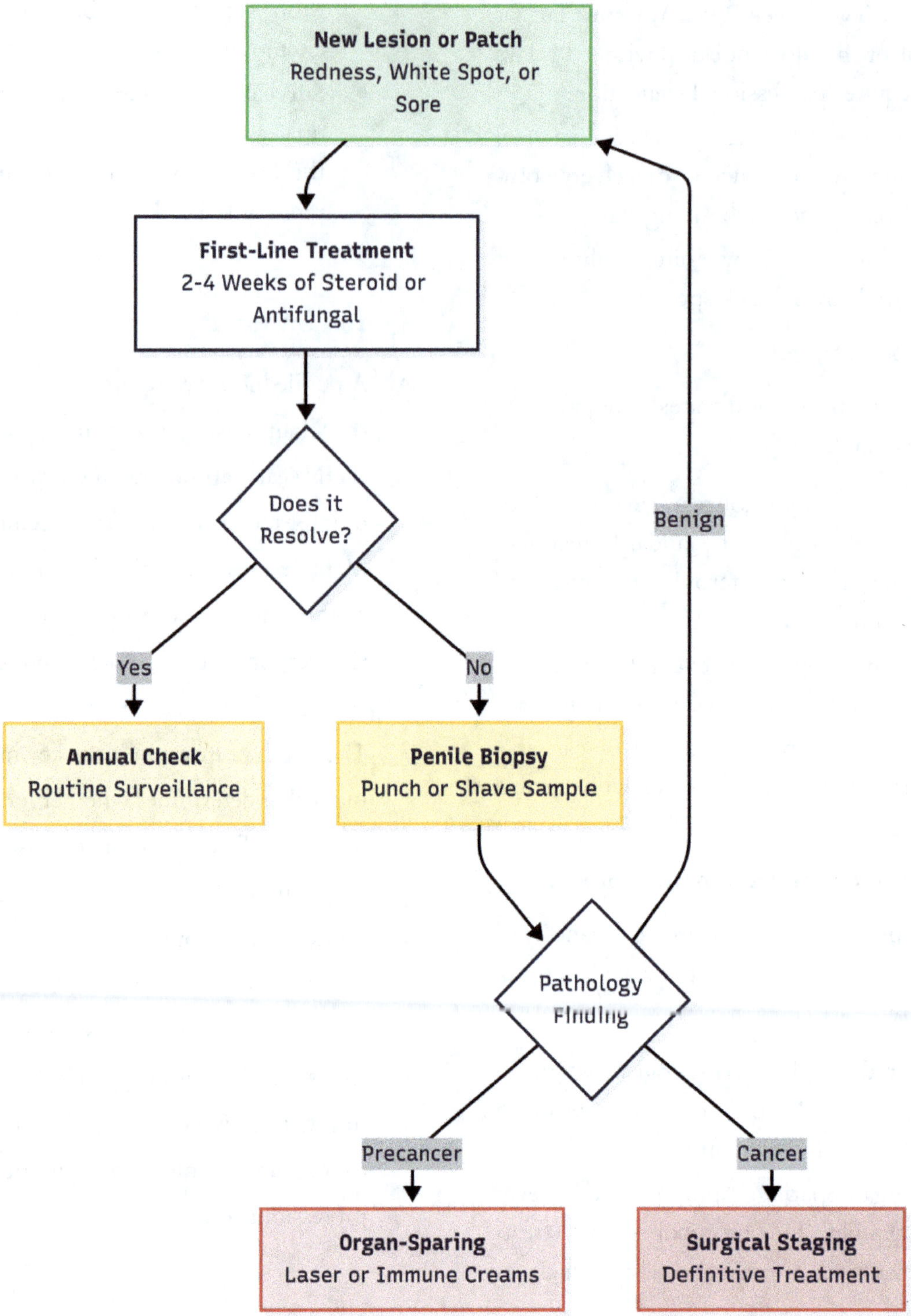
New Lesion or Patch
Redness, White Spot, or Sore
First-Line Treatment
2-4 Weeks of Steroid or Antifungal
Does it Resolve?
Yes
No
Annual Check
Routine Surveillance
Penile Biopsy
Punch or Shave Sample
Benign
Pathology Finding
Precancer
Cancer
Organ-Sparing
Laser or Immune Creams
Surgical Staging
Definitive Treatment

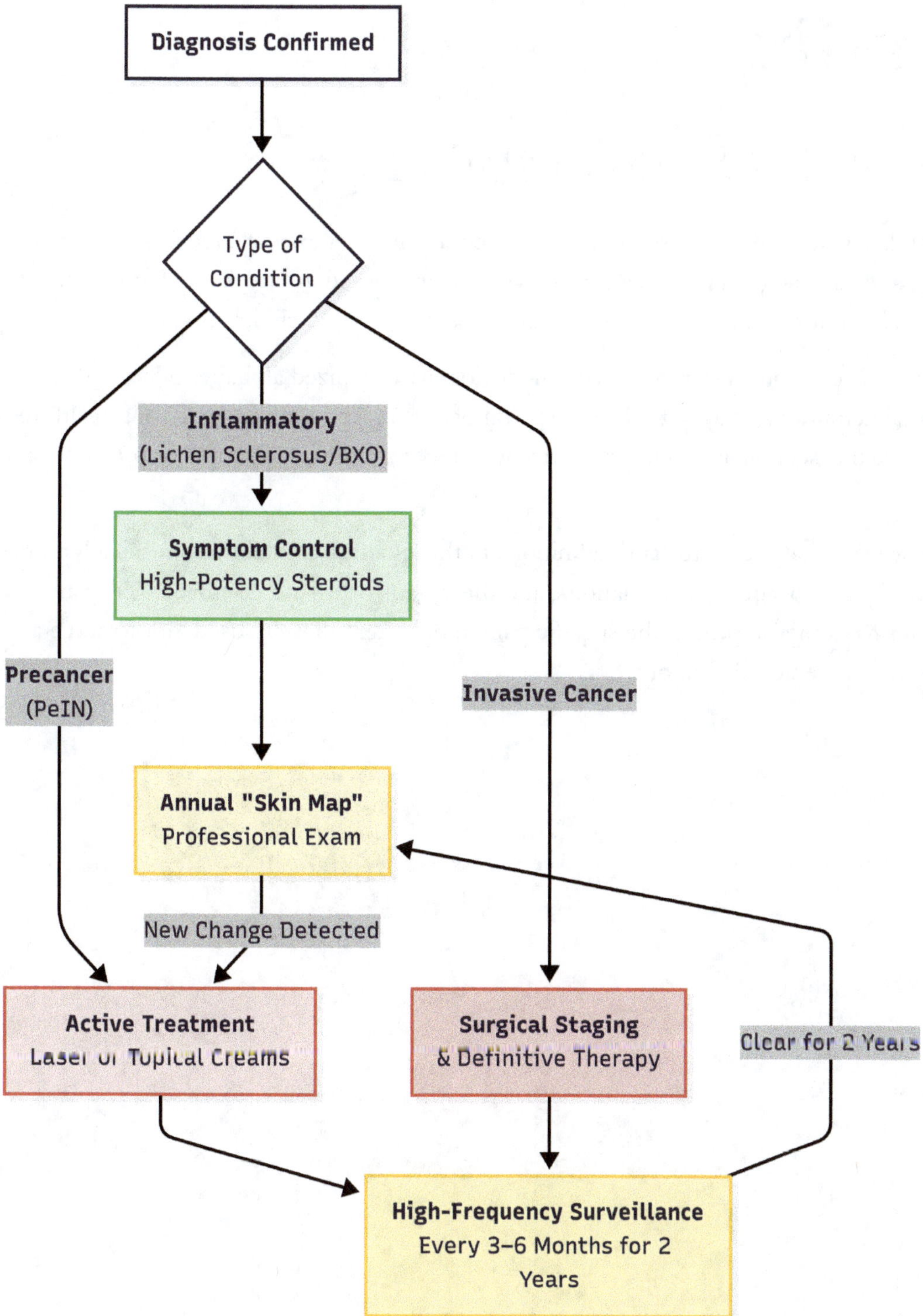
Diagnosis Confirmed
Type of Condition
Inflammatory (Lichen Sclerosus/BXO)
Symptom Control
High-Potency Steroids
Precancer (PeIN)
Invasive Cancer
Annual "Skin Map"
Professional Exam
New Change Detected
Active Treatment
Laser or Topical Creams
Surgical Staging
& Definitive Therapy
Clear for 2 Years
High-Frequency Surveillance
Every 3–6 Months for 2 Years

Appendix

Glossary of the World of Pathology

If you've ever felt like you needed a Rosetta Stone to decode your own medical records, you're not alone. Medicine, and pathology in particular, uses a vocabulary rooted in Greek and Latin, created for scientific precision but often forming an unintended barrier between clinicians and patients.

In this final chapter, you'll find a clear, patient-friendly glossary organized alphabetically. These aren't just technical definitions; they're tools to help you better understand the story your health records are telling. Use this section as a quick reference whenever you review a report or prepare for a follow-up visit.

Keep in mind, however, that the words and definitions in this glossary are tailored specifically to the context of this book, its procedures, explanations, and the organs or tissues discussed. They are meant to clarify terms as they appear in the specific paragraph where they are used, not to serve as exhaustive or universal medical definitions.

Glossary

10% Neutral Buffered Formalin: The standard chemical solution used to fix or preserve biopsy tissue, preventing decay by locking proteins in place.

24-Hour Urine Collection: A diagnostic procedure where a patient collects every drop of urine voided over a full day and night into a specialized container. In a parathyroid or kidney workup, this allows doctors to measure the total amount of calcium, creatinine, or protein excreted, providing a more accurate big picture of organ function than a single, one-time sample.

4-Week Rule (Bladder): A clinical protocol where a red, irritated patch in the bladder is treated for infection first; if it does not resolve within a month, a biopsy is triggered to rule out flat cancer (CIS).

4D-CT Scan: A high-speed imaging technique that uses time-sequenced contrast mapping to track the blood-flow patterns of tissues, helping doctors distinguish between normal structures and abnormal growths throughout the body.

4Kscore / PHI (Prostate Health Index): Advanced blood tests used as a second opinion when a PSA is elevated to help determine if a prostate biopsy is truly necessary.

ABCDE Rule: A mnemonic used to guide skin self-exams (Asymmetry, Border, Color, Diameter, Evolving).

Absolute Alcohol: High-purity (100%) ethanol. It is used in the dehydration stage of tissue processing to remove all traces of water from a specimen.

Accessioning: The critical first step in the laboratory where specimens are received, verified against doctor's orders, and assigned a unique tracking barcode.

ACS (American Cancer Society): A nationwide voluntary health organization dedicated to eliminating cancer.

Actinic Keratosis (AK): A rough, scaly patch on the skin caused by years of sun exposure; it is considered precancerous because it can develop into squamous cell carcinoma.

Active Surveillance: A treatment plan for low-risk cancer (common in prostate and sometimes early cervical changes) that involves close monitoring with regular tests and biopsies rather than immediate surgery or radiation.

Adenocarcinoma: A specific type of cancer that forms in glandular structures, such as the lining of the colon, lungs, or breast.

Adenocarcinoma (Lung): The most common type of lung cancer, usually starting in the mucus-producing glands in the outer parts of the lung.

Adenocarcinoma (Pancreas): The most common and aggressive form of pancreatic cancer, typically arising in the ducts that carry digestive juices.

Adenocarcinoma In Situ (AIS): A precancerous condition involving the glandular cells of the cervix; it requires careful management as it can be more difficult to track than surface cell changes.

Adenocarcinoma in Situ (Oral/Thyroid context): A localized, non-invasive cancer of the glandular tissues; in the thyroid, this is a critical distinction made to separate contained tumors from invasive ones.

Adenoma: A benign tag like growth made of glands. Example: A precancerous colon polyp. While not yet cancer, it has the potential to turn into cancer if left in the colon.

Adequacy (Endometrial biopsy and Cervical Pap Smear): A determination by the pathologist that enough tissue was collected during the biopsy to provide a reliable and definitive diagnosis.

AFP (Alpha-Fetoprotein): A blood marker used in liver protocols; elevated levels can signal the presence of liver cancer, especially in patients with known cirrhosis (scarring).

Alarm Symptoms: Specific red flag signs (like bleeding or unexplained weight loss) that mandate an immediate medical evaluation regardless of previous clear tests.

Anatomic Pathologist: A physician who studies the effects of disease on the body's organs and tissues through microscopic, chemical, and molecular examination.

Anatomic Pathology: The branch of medicine that involves the study of the effects of disease on the structure of body organs and tissues.

Anatomy: The branch of science concerned with the bodily structure of humans, animals, and other living organisms.

Angiomyolipoma: A common, benign (non-cancerous) tumor made up of fat, muscle, and blood vessels.

Animalcules: A historical term coined by Antonie van Leeuwenhoek to describe microscopic organisms, including bacteria and protozoa, seen under his early lenses.

ASCCP (American Society for Colposcopy and Cervical Pathology): The organization that provides guidelines for managing abnormal Pap smears and cervical biopsies.

ASCCP Guidelines: The professional standard of care protocols used by clinicians to decide exactly how to treat an abnormal Pap smear or cervical biopsy.

ASCUS / LSIL / HSIL: Terms used in Pap smear reports to describe abnormal cells; ASCUS is the mildest (uncertain), LSIL is low-grade, and HSIL is high-grade.

Aspirate (Bone Marrow): The liquid portion of the bone marrow removed during a biopsy; it allows pathologists to look at the fine details and shapes of individual developing blood cells.

ATA (American Thyroid Association): The leading organization focused on thyroid health and the management of thyroid nodules.

Atypia / Atypical: A yellow light term describing cells that look slightly abnormal or unusual under the microscope but are not yet clearly cancerous. In the uterus (endometrial atypia), it is a significant warning sign for potential cancer.

Atypical Ductal Hyperplasia (ADH): A high-risk breast condition where cells in the milk ducts look abnormal and are crowded, increasing the future risk of breast cancer.

Autopsy: The post-mortem examination of a body to discover the cause of death or the extent of disease.

Axilla: The medical term for the armpit; clinicians check the lymph nodes in this area during a professional breast exam.

Balanitis Xerotica Obliterans (BXO): Another name for Lichen Sclerosus when it affects the penis; it causes white, scarred patches that can lead to discomfort or urinary issues.

Barrett's Esophagus: A condition where the lining of the esophagus changes to resemble the lining of the intestine, usually caused by chronic acid reflux (GERD); it requires regular monitoring.

Basal Cell Carcinoma (BCC): The most common form of skin cancer. It grows slowly and rarely spreads to other parts of the body but can be locally destructive.

BCG (Bacillus Calmette-Guérin): A type of immunotherapy liquid placed directly into the bladder to help the immune system reach and kill surface-level cancer cells.

Benign: A term used to describe a tumor or growth that is not cancerous and does not spread to other parts of the body.

Bethesda System: The universal 1-through-6 grading scale used to report thyroid biopsy results. Category 2 is benign, while Category 6 is malignant.

BI-RADS (Breast Imaging-Reporting and Data System): A universal scoring system (0 - 6) used by radiologists to communicate how suspicious a breast finding is and what the next step should be.

Bile Duct Cancer (Cholangiocarcinoma): A type of cancer that originates in the tubes that carry bile from the liver to the gallbladder and small intestine.

Biomarker Testing (Lung): Specialized tests that look for genetic switches (like EGFR, ALK, or ROS1) in lung cancer cells; finding these allows patients to take targeted pills instead of traditional chemotherapy.

Biomarkers: Biological keys (like ER, PR, and HER2) found on cancer cells that tell doctors which specific drugs or therapies will be most effective.

Biopsy: The removal of a small piece of tissue from a living body for examination to determine the presence or extent of a disease.

Bios (Life) and Opsis (To See): The Greek etymological roots of the word biopsy.

BK Virus: A common virus that usually remains dormant but can become active and damage a transplanted kidney, often requiring a biopsy to diagnose.

Blasts: Immature baby blood cells. In a healthy bone marrow factory, these make up less than 5% of the population; a high percentage (over 20%) typically triggers a diagnosis of acute leukemia.

Blue Nevus: A type of benign (harmless) mole that appears blue or gray because the pigment-producing cells are located deep in the dermis.

Board-Certified: A designation for a physician who has passed a rigorous examination by a medical specialty board.

BPH (Benign Prostatic Hyperplasia): A common, non-cancerous enlargement of the prostate gland that can cause a rise in PSA levels and urinary symptoms.

BRCA / Lynch Syndrome: Genetic mutations that, while often associated with breast or colon cancer, also trigger a high-risk screening protocol for pancreatic cancer.

BRCA1 / BRCA2: Genetic mutations that significantly increase the lifetime risk of developing breast and ovarian cancer.

Breast MRI: A high-sensitivity imaging test using magnetic fields to create detailed pictures of breast tissue, often used for high-risk screening.

CA 19-9: A blood marker (liquid biopsy) often used alongside tissue biopsies to help monitor pancreatic cancer or support a diagnosis.

Calcifications: Tiny calcium deposits in the breast that show up as white spots on a mammogram; while often benign, certain patterns can signal early cancer (DCIS).

Capsule (Thyroid): The protective shell surrounding a thyroid nodule. Pathologists look to see if cells have broken through this shell to determine if a tumor is cancerous.

Carcinoma in Situ: Cancer that is at the earliest possible stage, where abnormal cells are present but have not yet spread into the surrounding healthy tissue.

Carcinoma in Situ (CIS) (Bladder): A flat, high-grade (aggressive) cancer that stays on the surface of the bladder lining but has a high risk of spreading if not treated.

Cassette: A small, rectangular, perforated plastic box used to hold and identify tissue samples during the chemical processing stages

CBC (Complete Blood Count): The standard first-line blood test that measures red cells, white cells, and platelets; abnormalities here often trigger the protocol for a bone marrow biopsy.

Celiac Disease: An immune reaction to eating gluten that creates a specific pattern of inflammation in the small intestine visible under a microscope.

Cell Block: A technique where cells from a needle biopsy are concentrated into a small paraffin block; this allows the pathologist to perform more advanced stains and molecular tests.

Cell Theory: The scientific theory that all living organisms are made up of cells, and that cells are the basic unit of structural and organizational life.

Chain of Custody: The rigorous process of tracking a specimen from the moment it leaves the patient's body to the final diagnosis to ensure it is never mislabeled or lost.

Chromatin: The material (DNA and proteins) inside the cell nucleus; pathologists look for clumpy or dark chromatin as a sign of cancer.

Chronic Pancreatitis: Long-term inflammation of the pancreas that can cause scarring (fibrosis) and occasionally mimic the appearance of a tumor on imaging.

CIN (Cervical Intraepithelial Neoplasia): A grading scale (1, 2, or 3) for abnormal cervical cells found on a biopsy. CIN 1 is mild/low-risk; CIN 3 is severe/precancerous.

Cirrhosis (F4 Fibrosis): The most advanced stage of liver scarring, where healthy tissue is replaced by scar tissue, blocking blood flow and impairing liver function.

Clear, Negative, or R0 Margins: A result indicating that no cancer cells were found at the very edge of the removed tissue, suggesting the entire tumor was captured.

Clearing: A step in tissue processing, usually using xylene, that removes alcohol from the tissue and makes it transparent (translucent) so it can be infiltrated with paraffin wax.

Clinical Breast Exam (CBE): A physical examination of the breast and underarm performed by a healthcare professional to feel for lumps or changes.

Clonal Process: A term used in lymph node pathology to describe a group of identical, abnormal cells that are multiplying out of control; this is a hallmark of lymphoma.

Colonoscopy: A procedure where a flexible camera is used to inspect the entire colon and remove polyps.

Colposcopy: A procedure where a doctor uses a magnifying lens (colposcope) and a mild vinegar solution to identify and biopsy abnormal areas on the cervix.

Concordant / Discordant: Terms used to describe whether the pathology result (the biology) matches the radiologist's suspicion (the imaging).

Core (Bone Marrow): A solid, slender cylinder of bone tissue removed during a biopsy; it shows the architecture and scaffolding of the marrow factory.

Core Needle Biopsy: A procedure using a hollow, spring-loaded needle to fire into a site and capture a solid cylinder (core) of tissue, allowing the pathologist to see the tissue architecture. Organ-specific versions are used for the breast, lung, and lymph nodes.

Creatinine / eGFR: Blood tests used to measure how well the kidneys are filtering waste; a rising creatinine or falling eGFR often triggers a kidney biopsy.

Crush Artifact: A technical limitation where the cells were squeezed or flattened during collection, making their internal details impossible to see under the microscope.

CT Scan (Computed Tomography): A medical imaging technique that uses computer-processed combinations of multiple X-ray measurements taken from different angles to produce tomographic images.

Cystitis Cystica: A common, benign inflammatory condition where small, fluid-filled pockets form in the lining of the bladder due to chronic irritation.

Cystoscopy: A procedure where a urologist uses a thin camera to look inside the bladder; it is the primary way bladder biopsies are performed.

Cytogenetics: A high-tech laboratory analysis of the chromosomes within marrow cells; this provides a genetic map to identify the specific subtype of a blood disorder.

Cytology / Cytopathology: The branch of pathology that studies individual cells (often from fluids or thin needle aspirations) rather than solid chunks of tissue.

D&C (Dilation and Curettage): A procedure to scrape and collect tissue from the inside of the uterus; used as additional layer of care if a standard biopsy is inconclusive.

Dehydration: A step in tissue processing that uses graduated concentrations of alcohol to remove all water from a specimen.

Dermatopathologist: A specialist in both dermatology (skin) and pathology who focuses on diagnosing skin diseases at a microscopic level.

Dermatopathology: The study of skin diseases at a microscopic and molecular level.

Dermatoscope: A handheld tool used by dermatologists that uses polarized light and magnification to see structures beneath the skin's surface.

Differential Diagnosis: The process of differentiating between two or more conditions which share similar symptoms. For a pathologist, it is an internal shortlist of possibilities (e.g., infection vs. tumor) used to guide testing.

Discordance: A red flag occurring when the biopsy says benign (normal) but the imaging or symptoms strongly suggest cancer; this usually triggers an automatic re-evaluation.

Ductal Carcinoma In Situ (DCIS): An early, non-invasive form of breast cancer where abnormal cells are found only inside the milk ducts and have not spread.

Dysplasia: The presence of abnormal-looking cells within a tissue, which may signify a stage preceding the development of cancer.

Dysplasia (Oral): Abnormal cell growth in the lining of the mouth, graded as mild, moderate, or severe. High-grade dysplasia is considered a true precancer.

EGD (Esophagogastroduodenoscopy): Also known as an Upper Endoscopy; a procedure to inspect the esophagus, stomach, and the first part of the small intestine.

Embedding: The stage where a histotechnologist places processed tissue into a mold and surrounds it with liquid paraffin wax, which then hardens into a solid block for slicing.

Endometrial Intraepithelial Neoplasia (EIN): A precancerous condition where the lining of the uterus is overgrown with abnormal cells; also known as atypical hyperplasia.

Endometrium: The specialized tissue that lines the inside of the uterus and thickens/sheds during the menstrual cycle.

Eosin: A pink acidic dye used in histological staining to highlight cytoplasm and connective tissue.

Epidermal Inclusion Cyst: A common, non-cancerous bump beneath the skin filled with keratin (skin protein).

Epithelium vs. Dermis (Penile): The two main layers examined in a penile biopsy. The epithelium is the surface layer where precancer (PeIN) sits, while the dermis is the deeper tissue where invasive cancer roots.

Estrogen / Progesterone Receptors (ER/PR): Proteins on breast cancer cells that catch hormones; if positive, the cancer can be treated with hormone-blocking medications.

EUS (Endoscopic Ultrasound): The standard of care procedure for pancreatic biopsies; a scope with an ultrasound tip is passed into the stomach to look through the stomach wall and guide a needle into the pancreas.

Excisional Biopsy (Lymph Node): A minor surgical procedure to remove an entire lymph node; this is often the standard of care for diagnosing lymphoma because the pathologist needs to see the node's complete internal architecture.

FASCP / FASDP / FCAP: Professional fellowships indicating a physician is a member of the American Society for Clinical Pathology, the American Society of Dermatopathology, or the College of American Pathologists.

Fibroadenoma: A very common, benign (non-cancerous) breast tumor made of both glandular and connective tissue.

FibroScan: A specialized, non-invasive ultrasound that measures the stiffness of the liver to determine the level of scarring (fibrosis) without needing a needle.

Fibrosis (F0 - F4): The medical term for scarring. In the liver, it is graded from F0 (no scarring) to F4 (cirrhosis). In the bone marrow, it refers to a toughening of the marrow space that hinders cell production.

Fine Needle Aspiration (FNA): A diagnostic technique using a very thin, hollow needle to investigate lumps or nodules by withdrawing (aspirating) individual cells or fluid.

Fixation: The chemical process (usually using formalin) that freezes the biological state of cells, stopping them from breaking down or rotting.

Flow Cytometry: A high-tech laboratory test that uses lasers to analyze the fingerprint of markers on individual cells; used to identify specific types of leukemia and lymphoma.

FNA / FNB (Fine Needle Aspiration/Biopsy): The two types of needle sampling used during an EUS; FNA collects individual cells, while FNB collects small pieces of intact tissue.

Focal / Foci: A term meaning the disease is only in small, isolated islands. If a needle misses these tiny islands, it results in a false negative.

Formalin (Formaldehyde): A chemical fixative used to preserve biological tissues by preventing decay and fixing proteins in place.

Frozen Section: A rapid diagnostic procedure performed while a patient is undergoing surgery; tissue is frozen quickly to allow for immediate microscopic examination and surgical guidance.

Fukuoka Guidelines: The international medical protocol used to decide whether a pancreatic cyst is low risk (monitor with scans) or high risk (requires surgery).

Gastrointestinal and Hepatopathology: The study of diseases of the digestive tract and the liver.

General Practitioner: A medical doctor who treats acute and chronic illnesses and provides preventive care and health education to patients.

Gleason System / Gleason Score: The primary grading scale for prostate cancer aggressiveness. It ranges from 6 (low-grade) to 8 - 10 (aggressive).

Glomeruli: The tiny, microscopic filters in the kidney that clean the blood. A high-quality kidney biopsy usually needs to contain at least 10 of these for an accurate diagnosis.

Grade: A measurement of how wild or aggressive cancer cells look; low-grade cells look mostly normal, while high-grade cells look chaotic.

Grade Group (Prostate): A simplified 1 - 5 scale based on the Gleason score. Grade Group 1 is the least aggressive; Grade Group 5 is the most aggressive.

Granuloma: A small area of inflammation in the lung or lymph node, often caused by an old infection (like a scar) rather than cancer.

Grossing / Gross Room: The area of the lab where specimens are examined with the naked eye, described, measured, and sometimes inked for orientation before being cut into smaller pieces for processing.

GU (Genitourinary) Pathology: The study of diseases of the urinary tract and the male reproductive system.

H. pylori (Helicobacter pylori): A spiral-shaped bacterium that lives in the stomach and can cause ulcers and chronic inflammation.

H&E (Hematoxylin and Eosin): The standard stain used in histology. Hematoxylin stains cell nuclei blue/purple, and Eosin stains other structures (like cytoplasm and collagen) pink.

HCC (Hepatocellular Carcinoma): The most common form of primary liver cancer, usually developing in the setting of chronic liver disease or cirrhosis.

Hematoxylin: A natural dye used in histology to stain the nuclei of cells a deep blue or purple.

Hematuria: The medical term for blood in the urine.

HER2 (Human Epidermal Growth Factor Receptor 2): A protein that can promote the growth of cancer cells; knowing if a tumor is HER2-positive allows for targeted treatment.

Heterogeneity / Heterogeneous: A state where a tumor is diverse in content; some areas may be aggressive while others are quiet or benign. This often necessitates multiple samples.

High-Grade: A term describing cancer cells that look very different from normal cells and tend to grow and spread more quickly.

High-Grade Dysplasia (GI): Advanced cellular changes in a polyp that indicate a high risk of turning into invasive cancer.

Hilum (Lymph Node): The fatty center of a lymph node where blood vessels enter and exit. In a healthy node, this is visible on ultrasound; if it disappears, the node is considered suspicious.

Histology: The study of the microscopic structure of tissues.

Histopathology: The microscopic examination of tissue in order to study the manifestations of disease.

Histotechnologist: A medical professional who processes and prepares very thin slices of human tissue onto glass slides for a pathologist to examine.

Hodgkin vs. Non-Hodgkin Lymphoma: Two broad categories of cancer that start in the lymph nodes. They look different under the microscope and require different treatment strategies.

Hormone Replacement Therapy (HRT): Medications containing female hormones used to replace those the body no longer makes after menopause.

Hot Nodule: A thyroid nodule that produces excess thyroid hormone (detected on a nuclear scan). These are almost always benign and rarely require a biopsy.

HPV (Human Papillomavirus): A very common virus; certain high-risk strains are the primary cause of cervical precancer and cancer.

Hypercalcemia: Elevated calcium levels in the blood; this is the primary clinical trigger for a parathyroid workup, often discovered during routine blood tests.

Hypercellular vs. Hypocellular: Terms describing the crowdedness of the bone marrow. Hypercellular means the factory is over-crowded; Hypocellular means it is under-producing.

Hyperplasia: An overgrowth of cells. In the uterus, it can range from benign thickening to precancerous. In the parathyroid, it refers to all four glands becoming enlarged.

Hyperplastic Polyp: A very common type of colon polyp that is typically benign and has a very low risk of turning into cancer.

Hyperthyroidism: A condition where the thyroid gland is overactive, often signaled by a low TSH (Thyroid Stimulating Hormone) level.

IFTA (Interstitial Fibrosis and Tubular Atrophy): A term used in kidney pathology reports to describe the amount of permanent scarring versus active, treatable inflammation.

IgA Nephropathy: A common kidney disease that occurs when an antibody called IgA builds up in the kidneys, causing inflammation.

IHC (Immunohistochemistry): A laboratory method that uses antibodies to check for certain markers (antigens) in tissue, helping to identify the specific type or origin of cancer.

Immunotherapy: A type of cancer treatment that helps your own immune system recognize and attack cancer cells; biopsies often test for markers like PD-L1 to see if this will work.

In-Situ vs. Invasive (Penile): In-situ means abnormal cells are sitting only on the surface; Invasive means they have broken through the boundary into deeper tissue.

Inadequate / Insufficient / Scant: These all mean the same thing, there wasn't enough material in the sample to make a reliable diagnosis.

Indeterminate (Bethesda Category 3 or 4): A result where thyroid cells look unusual but the pathologist cannot say for sure if they are cancerous without surgery or molecular testing.

Infiltration: The stage in tissue processing where warm liquid paraffin wax fills the microscopic spaces in the tissue once water and alcohol have been removed.

Interventional Radiology (IR): A medical sub-specialty that uses real-time imaging (like CT or Ultrasound) to guide needles deep into the body with high precision.

Intravesical Therapy: Any treatment where liquid medication (chemotherapy or immunotherapy) is put directly into the bladder through a catheter.

Invasion: The process where cancer cells push through their natural boundaries into the surrounding healthy scaffolding of the body.

Invasive Ductal Carcinoma (IDC): The most common type of breast cancer, which begins in the milk ducts and invades the surrounding breast tissue.

Invasive Lobular Carcinoma (ILC): A type of breast cancer that begins in the milk-producing glands (lobules) of the breast.

IPMN (Intraductal Papillary Mucinous Neoplasm): A specific type of pancreatic cyst that produces mucus; because these can sometimes turn into cancer, they follow a strict surveillance protocol.

Iron Stores: A specific measurement taken during a bone marrow biopsy to see how much raw material (iron) is available for making new red blood cells.

Jaundice: A yellowing of the skin and eyes often caused by a pancreatic mass blocking the bile duct; this is a common trigger for an urgent diagnostic workup.

LDCT (Low-Dose Computed Tomography): A special, low-radiation X-ray used for annual lung cancer screening in high-risk individuals (smokers or former smokers).

LEEP (Loop Electrosurgical Excision Procedure): A treatment that uses a thin wire loop with an electric current to remove abnormal (precancerous) cervical tissue.

Leukoplakia: A thickened, white patch on the gums, tongue, or inside of the cheeks that cannot be scraped off; it can sometimes be precancerous.

Lichen Planus: A chronic inflammatory condition that can cause lacy white patches or sores inside the mouth; it is benign but requires monitoring.

Lichen Sclerosus: A chronic inflammatory skin condition of the vulva that causes thinning, whitening (like cigarette paper), and intense itching; it is benign but requires long-term management.

Lichen Sclerosus (Penile): A chronic inflammatory skin condition that causes thinning and whitening of the tissue; while benign, it requires long-term steroid treatment to prevent scarring and reduce cancer risk.

Liquid Biopsy: A test done on a sample of blood to look for cancer cells or circulating DNA from a tumor.

Lobules (Liver): The microscopic functional units of the liver, typically hexagonal in shape.

Local Anesthetic: A medication used to numb a specific, small area of the body (e.g., lidocaine) so the patient does not feel sharp pain during a biopsy.

Lumpectomy: A surgical procedure to remove a suspicious lump or known cancer from the breast while leaving the rest of the breast intact.

Lung-RADS: A standardized scoring system (1 - 4) used by radiologists to categorize lung nodules and determine how often they need to be scanned or if they need a biopsy.

Lymphocytes and Neutrophils: Types of white blood cells that represent the body's police force; their presence often indicates inflammation or infection.

Lymphoma: A type of cancer that begins in the cells of the immune system (lymphocytes) within the lymph nodes.

Lynch Syndrome: An inherited genetic condition that significantly increases the risk of several types of cancer, particularly colon and endometrial cancer.

Malignant: A term used to describe a tumor that is cancerous, meaning it can invade nearby tissue and spread to other parts of the body.

Mammogram: A low-dose X-ray of the breast used to detect tumors or calcifications.

Margins: The edges of a surgically removed piece of tissue.

MASLD (Metabolic Dysfunction-Associated Steatotic Liver Disease): The modern term for fatty liver associated with metabolic issues like diabetes or high cholesterol.

Melanoma: The most serious form of skin cancer, arising from pigment-producing cells (melanocytes). The pathology report will measure its Breslow Thickness (depth).

Merkel Cell Carcinoma: A very rare but highly aggressive skin cancer that can sometimes be mistaken for a harmless cyst to the naked eye.

Metastasis: The spread of cancer cells from the place where they first formed to another part of the body.

Metastatic Cancer: Cancer that started in one organ (like the breast or colon) and has traveled through the highway of the lymph system to a lymph node.

Metastatic Liver Disease: Cancer that started in another organ (like the colon or breast) and traveled to the liver; this is the most common type of liver mass.

Micron (um): A unit of length equal to one-millionth of a meter. Tissue slices are typically cut at 4 microns thick, while a human hair is about 70 microns wide.

Microtome: A specialized precision instrument used to cut extremely thin slices of material (usually tissue embedded in wax) for microscopic examination.

Minimal Change Disease: A kidney condition that causes large amounts of protein to leak into the urine; it is called minimal change because the damage is only visible under an electron microscope.

Mitosis / Mitotic Figure: The process of a cell physically dividing into two; seeing many of these figures suggests a tumor is growing rapidly.

Mohs Surgery: A precise surgical technique used for some skin cancers where thin layers of skin are removed and examined immediately under a microscope until only cancer-free tissue remains.

Molecular Testing (Thyroid): Advanced genetic testing performed on biopsy cells to look for specific mutations (like BRAF or RAS) to clarify an indeterminate result.

MRI (Magnetic Resonance Imaging): A medical imaging technique used in radiology to form pictures of the anatomy and the physiological processes of the body using strong magnetic fields.

MRI-Fusion Biopsy: A high-tech procedure where a previous MRI scan is digitally fused with a live ultrasound to help the urologist aim the biopsy needle at a specific suspicious spot.

Muscle Invasive Bladder Cancer: A stage of cancer where the cells have grown into the thick muscle wall of the bladder, requiring more intensive treatment like surgery or radiation.

Myelodysplastic Syndrome (MDS): A group of disorders where the bone marrow does not produce enough healthy, mature blood cells; often referred to as bone marrow failure.

NASH / MASH: Terms for metabolic-associated steatohepatitis (fatty liver disease with inflammation), which may require a liver biopsy to determine the extent of scarring.

Neuroendocrine Tumor (NET): A less common type of pancreatic tumor that grows from hormone-producing cells; these typically grow slower and have a different treatment path than adenocarcinoma.

Neuropathology: The study of disease of nervous system tissue.

NIDDK (National Institute of Diabetes and Digestive and Kidney Diseases): A branch of the NIH that provides data and research on digestive and kidney health.

Non-Diagnostic / Nondiagnostic: A catch-all result meaning not enough cells were collected to provide a definitive answer, usually requiring a repeat procedure.

Non-Muscle Invasive Bladder Cancer: Cancer cells that are confined to the inner lining of the bladder and have not yet reached the muscle layer.

Nottingham Grade: A specific grading system used to categorize the aggressiveness of breast cancer.

Nucleus / Nucleus (Cellular): The command center of a cell containing its genetic material; pathologists check its size, shape, and internal details to determine if a cell is healthy or diseased.

On-Site Assessment (ROSE): A process where a scientist or pathologist checks the needle sample during the procedure to ensure enough cells were captured before the patient goes home.

Oncocytoma: A benign (non-cancerous) kidney tumor that can look very similar to cancer on a CT scan, often requiring a biopsy to tell them apart.

Open Biopsy: A traditional surgical procedure where a large incision is made under general anesthesia to remove a tissue sample; largely replaced by needle biopsies today.

Organ-Sparing Approach: A treatment philosophy (using creams, lasers, or limited surgery) aimed at removing diseased penile tissue while preserving as much healthy function and appearance as possible.

Pack-Year: A way to measure smoking history; it is calculated by multiplying the number of packs smoked per day by the number of years smoked.

Papillary Thyroid Carcinoma: The most common type of thyroid cancer; it is typically slow-growing and has an exceptionally high cure rate.

Papillary vs. Sessile (Bladder): Terms describing the shape of a growth; Papillary growths look like small ferns or broccoli on a stalk, while Sessile growths are flat against the bladder wall.

Paraffin Wax: A white or colorless soft solid used in pathology to infiltrate and surround tissue specimens to provide support for thin slicing.

Parathyroid Adenoma: A benign (non-cancerous) tumor of one of the parathyroid glands that causes it to overproduce hormone and raise blood calcium levels.

Parathyroid Hormone (PTH): The hormone responsible for regulating calcium. It is often measured directly from a biopsy needle (PTH Washout) to confirm the tissue's identity.

Pathologist: A physician who interprets and diagnoses the changes caused by disease in tissues and body fluids.

Pathologist's Eye: A metaphorical term for the trained ability of a pathologist to recognize complex patterns and cellular abnormalities quickly.

Pathologists' Assistant: A highly trained professional who performs the initial examination and dissection (grossing) of surgical specimens.

Pathology: The science of the causes and effects of diseases, especially the branch of medicine that deals with the laboratory examination of samples.

Pathology Informatics: A subspecialty of pathology that focuses on the management and analysis of health and biomedical data.

PAX8: A protein marker used in special staining to identify if a cell originated in the kidney, thyroid, or female reproductive tract.

PCOS (Polycystic Ovary Syndrome): A hormonal disorder that can cause a buildup of the uterine lining, increasing the risk of hyperplasia.

PeIN (Penile Intraepithelial Neoplasia): A precancerous change in the skin cells of the penis. It is highly treatable if caught before it becomes invasive.

Perineural Invasion: A general finding where cancer cells are seen wrapping around or hitching a ride on a nerve.

Perineural Invasion (Prostate): A finding where cancer cells are seen touching or surrounding the small nerves near the prostate; while noted in the report, it doesn't always change the cancer stage.

Peripheral Smear: A test where a drop of blood is spread on a slide and examined; it is the scouting report done before a bone marrow biopsy.

PI-RADS (Prostate Imaging-Reporting and Data System): A 1 - 5 scoring system used by radiologists to describe how likely a spot on a prostate MRI is to be significant for cancer.

Pipelle: A thin, flexible plastic tube used to perform an endometrial biopsy in a doctor's office using light suction.

Pneumothorax: A potential complication of a lung biopsy where air leaks out of the lung and into the chest cavity.

Polarity (Cellular): The organized up and down orientation of cells; a loss of polarity is a sign of chaotic, potentially cancerous growth.

Positive Margins: A result indicating that cancer cells reach the very edge of the removed specimen, meaning some cancer may still be left in the patient.

PPE (Personal Protective Equipment): Protective clothing or equipment designed to protect the wearer from injury or the spread of infection.

Precision Medicine: A medical model that customizes healthcare, with treatments tailored to the individual based on their genetic or protein signature.

Primary Hyperparathyroidism: A condition where one or more parathyroid glands produce too much PTH, leading to high blood calcium and kidney stones.

Prosector's Paronychia: A historical term for an infection of the hands contracted by pathologists or students during autopsies.

Prostatitis: Inflammation or infection of the prostate gland, which can cause pain and temporarily high PSA levels.

PSA (Prostate-Specific Antigen): A protein made by the prostate; elevated levels in the blood can signal cancer, but also BPH or infection.

PSMA-PET Scan: A specialized imaging test used to see if prostate cancer cells have traveled to other parts of the body.

Pulmonary Pathology: The study of diseases of the lungs and thoracic cavity.

Pulmonologist: A doctor who specializes in the respiratory system and often performs biopsies from inside the lung using a scope.

Punch Biopsy: A tool that works like a tiny, circular cookie cutter to take a deep, cylindrical core of skin.

Radiology-Pathology Correlation: The safety process where the doctor double-checks that the pathology result actually fits what was seen on the imaging.

Reactive / Inflammatory: A diagnosis meaning the tissue is reacting to injury, infection, or allergy rather than being cancerous.

Reactive Lymph Node: A very common, non-cancerous finding where a lymph node is swollen because it is actively fighting an infection or responding to inflammation.

Renal Cell Carcinoma (RCC): The most common type of kidney cancer, which begins in the lining of the small tubes inside the kidney.

Renal Pathology: A subspecialty of anatomic pathology that deals with the diagnosis of medical diseases of the kidneys.

Resectable: A surgical term meaning a tumor is positioned in a way that it can be safely and completely removed by a surgeon.

Residency: A stage of graduate medical training where a doctor practices medicine under the supervision of fully licensed physicians.

Seeding: The rare concern that a biopsy needle might drag cancer cells along its path; modern techniques make this extremely unlikely.

Sepsis: A life-threatening reaction to an infection that can cause widespread inflammation and organ failure.

Sessile: A term describing a growth that is flat or broad-based, rather than being on a stalk.

Sessile Serrated Lesion (SSL): A type of precancerous polyp that is often flat and can be harder to detect during a colonoscopy than a typical stalk polyp.

Sestamibi (Technetium sestamibi): A radiopharmaceutical agent used in nuclear medicine imaging to visualize the heart, parathyroid glands, and breast tissue.

Sestamibi Scan: A nuclear medicine test where overactive parathyroid glands light up, helping the surgeon find the exact location of the problem.

Shave Biopsy: A technique using a small blade to shave off the top layers of a skin growth.

Social Distancing (Cellular): A metaphorical term for the healthy space and boundaries cells normally maintain between each other.

Specimen Inking: The application of colored dyes to the outside of a tissue sample to help the pathologist identify the top, bottom, or edges under the microscope.

Specimen X-ray: A safety step used during breast biopsies to confirm that the target (like calcium spots) is actually inside the tissue cores before they are sent to the lab.

Squamous Cell Carcinoma (Lung): A type of lung cancer that usually begins in the larger breathing tubes (bronchi) in the center of the chest.

Squamous Cell Carcinoma (Oral): The most common type of oral cancer, arising from the flat cells that line the mouth and lips.

Squamous Cell Carcinoma (Penile): The most common type of penile cancer, often linked to long-term inflammation or certain types of HPV.

Squamous Cell Carcinoma (SCC): The second most common skin cancer; it arises from the outer layer of the skin and has a higher risk of spreading than basal cell carcinoma.

Stereotactic Targeting: A high-precision biopsy method using computers and X-rays to find a target that is too small to be seen or felt by hand.

Surgical Pathology: The study of tissues removed during a surgical procedure to help diagnose a disease and determine a treatment plan.

Suture: A stitch or row of stitches holding together the edges of a wound or surgical incision.

Symmetry Check: A clinical protocol in oral exams where the provider compares one side of the mouth to the other to identify unusual, one-sided spots.

Synoptic Report: A standardized, checklist-style summary at the end of a pathology report that provides essential data points for the surgical team.

Tamoxifen: A medication used to treat or prevent breast cancer; it can sometimes cause the uterine lining to thicken as a side effect.

TBSE (Total Body Skin Exam): A professional head-to-toe check performed by a clinician to look for suspicious spots.

Test of Cure: Follow-up testing performed after a procedure (like a LEEP) to ensure all abnormal cells were successfully addressed.

Three-Week Rule (Lymph Nodes): A clinical protocol where doctors monitor a swollen node for 21 days; if it doesn't shrink after a virus passes, a biopsy is typically ordered.

TI-RADS (Thyroid Imaging Reporting and Data System): A scoring system used by radiologists to rate thyroid nodules on an ultrasound to determine if a biopsy is needed.

Tissue Architecture: The physical arrangement and neighborhood of cells; how they sit next to each other in the tissue.

Tissue Marker (Clip): A tiny metal object placed at the biopsy site to mark the spot for future imaging or surgery.

Trans-perineal Biopsy: A prostate biopsy where the needle enters through the skin between the scrotum and anus, offering a lower infection risk.

Transformation Zone: The specific area on the cervix (or in the oral cavity) where two types of cells meet; this is the most common site for abnormal changes to begin.

Transrectal Biopsy: The traditional method for a prostate biopsy where the needle passes through the rectal wall.

Transvaginal Ultrasound: An imaging test used to measure the thickness of the uterine lining; a thickness over 4mm in postmenopausal women often triggers a biopsy.

Transvenous (Transjugular) Biopsy: A specialized liver biopsy where the needle reaches the liver through the veins to minimize bleeding risk in high-risk patients.

Trichrome Stained: A specialized staining method used to distinguish between muscle fibers and connective tissue (fibrosis).

TSH (Thyroid Stimulating Hormone): A blood test that measures thyroid function; it is a standard part of evaluating any thyroid lump.

Tubular Adenoma: The most common type of precancerous colon polyp.

TURBT (Transurethral Resection of Bladder Tumor): A procedure to both biopsy and remove a bladder tumor using a scope passed through the urethra.

Two-Week Rule (Penile / Vulvar): A critical safety protocol stating that any sore, ulcer, or cut that does not heal within 14 days must be professionally evaluated and potentially biopsied.

UACR (Urine Albumin-to-Creatinine Ratio): A urine test used to detect small amounts of protein leaking from the kidney filters, serving as an early warning of damage.

USMLE (United States Medical Licensing Examination): A three-step examination for medical licensure in the United States.

Vacuum-Assisted Needle Biopsy: A procedure that uses a vacuum-powered instrument to collect multiple tissue samples through a single small incision.

VELscope: A specialized blue-light tool used by dentists to detect abnormal oral tissue not visible under normal light.

VIN (Vulvar Intraepithelial Neoplasia): A precancerous change where abnormal cells are found on the surface of the vulvar skin, graded 1, 2, or 3 based on severity.

Washout (PTH): A technique where the saline used to rinse a biopsy needle is tested for hormone concentration to confirm the tissue is parathyroid.

Well-Differentiated: Cells that still look very much like the healthy tissue they came from; usually a sign of a less aggressive tumor.

WSI (Whole Slide Imaging): The process of scanning glass slides to create high-resolution digital images for diagnosis.

X-ray: A form of high-energy electromagnetic radiation used to create images of the inside of the body.

Acknowledgments

The practice of pathology is a master - apprentice craft. No diagnostic skill is acquired in isolation, and every judgment I make today carries the imprint of mentors who sat beside me at the microscope, challenged my thinking, and modeled what diagnostic integrity truly means. This book reflects the collective wisdom, patience, and generosity of those teachers.

Residency at Hahnemann University Hospital

I am profoundly grateful to **Dr. Cheryl A. Hanau**, an extraordinary mentor and educator, for bringing me into the pathology residency program and providing the foundation upon which my career was built. I owe special thanks to **Dr. James England** for his leadership and mentorship as Chair.

My formative years were shaped by the guidance of **Dr. Corrado Minimo**, whose mentorship and humane leadership were invaluable. I also thank **Dr. Robert Ownbey**, **Dr. Steve Hou**, and **Dr. Fernando U. Garcia** for their early guidance and academic rigor.

I respectfully honor the memory of **Dr. Marian Haber**, whose lessons in surgical pathology endure in my daily practice. I am also indebted to **Dr. Suganthi Soundararajan** (surgical pathology), **Dr. Sydney Croul** (neuropathology), **Dr. Nedjema Sustento-Reodica**(renal pathology), and **Dr. Xiaoli Chen** (cytopathology), as well as **Dr. Vanlila K. Swami**, **Dr. Manjula Balasubramanian**, and **Dr. Christopher L. Emery**, whose collective mentorship and clinical excellence were instrumental to my growth. I honor the memory of **Dr. Fred Kayne** whose guidance in clinical chemistry will always be remembered.

Surgical Pathology at the Hospital of the University of Pennsylvania

I am deeply indebted to the faculty of the **Department of Pathology at the Hospital of the University of Pennsylvania**, whose diagnostic standards further sharpened my approach to complex disease. I extend my sincere thanks to **Dr. John E. Tomaszewski** for his guidance in GU and renal pathology, and to **Dr. Antonia R. Sepulveda** for her leadership and mentorship in surgical pathology.

I honor the enduring legacy of **Dr. Virginia A. LiVolsi**, whose transformative influence in gynecologic, thyroid, and surgical pathology left an indelible mark on my career. I am also grateful to **Dr. David E. Elder** for his mentorship in dermatopathology and gynecologic pathology, and to **Dr. Xiaowei (George) Xu** for his expertise in dermatopathology and surgical pathology.

My thanks also go to **Dr. Emma Elizabeth (Beth) Furth**, **Dr. Michael Feldman**, **Dr. Kathleen T. Montone**, **Dr. Leslie A. Litzky**, and **Dr. Priti Lal**, whose mentorship across subspecialties greatly expanded my diagnostic breadth.

Dermatopathology (Hahnemann and Dermpath Diagnostics)

Dermatopathology demands a unique analytical precision, and I was privileged to train under masters of the field. I am sincerely thankful to **Dr. Herbert B. Allen** for welcoming me into his fellowship program and to **Dr. Carrie Ann Cusack** for her dedicated mentorship.

I am deeply grateful to **Dr. Gary R. Kantor** and **Dr. Richard L. Spielvogel** for their unwavering support and personal mentorship. I also thank **Dr. Kenneth S. Resnik, Dr. Mario DiLeonardo,** and **Dr. Michael Kramer** for the invaluable insights they shared throughout my training.

Colleagues and Collaborators

I extend heartfelt appreciation to my residency senior colleagues, particularly **Dr. Mandana Mahmoodi, Dr. Sadia Salim, Dr. Todd Vinovrski,** and **Dr. Bethany Mapow**, for their collegiality and shared commitment to excellence. I also thank my fellow residents, including **Dr. Sarat Khandavalli, Dr. Lisa Chanal-Peddinghaus, Dr. Lisa Veith-Stevens, Dr. Bela Dalwadi, Dr. Marlon Osbourne, Dr. Essel Dulaimi Al-Saleem, Dr. Shuko Harada,** and **Dr. Melissa Munoz-Bishop**, for their camaraderie during our formative years.

A Final Note

Many mentors, fellows, and colleagues who profoundly influenced my development are not named here, but their guidance remains inseparable from my work. To the countless educators who shared diagnostic pearls at the multi-headed microscope: your lessons live on in every case I sign out.

Finally, I acknowledge with deep respect the **laboratory staff, histotechnologists, and pathologists' assistants**. Your technical excellence and quiet precision form the backbone of diagnostic medicine. This book is a tribute to the collaborative spirit of pathology and to those who practice it with integrity, rigor, and humility.

www.ingramcontent.com/pod-product-compliance
Lightning Source LLC
LaVergne TN
LVHW080046210926
848481LV00011B/3287